WHOLISTIC H
AND
LIVING YOGA

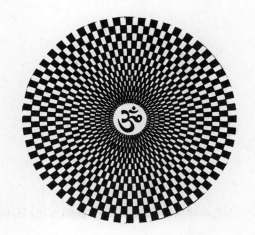

by
Malcolm Strutt

WHOLISTIC HEALTH AND LIVING YOGA

First Edition 1976
Second Edition
  First Printing 1977
  Second Printing 1979

Cover design and photography: John Hills   Cover model: Shelley Pallanes

Printed in the United States
by Kingsport Press

Library of Congress Cataloging in Publication Data

Strutt, Malcolm, 1936-
  Wholistic Health and Living Yoga.

  Includes index.
  1. Yoga, Hatha.   2. Yoga.   3. Mind and body.
I. Title.
RA781.7.S77   613.7   77-85790
ISBN 0-916438-08-2

UNIVERSITY OF THE TREES PRESS
P.O. BOX 644
BOULDER CREEK, CALIFORNIA 95006

Centre House 10a Airlie Gardens London W8 7AL

PREFACE

by

Christopher Hills

It is rare to find people who intuitively know that the Nuclear Evolution theory of the human personality is indeed the product of many years of study of Yoga, and it is truly gratifying for me, as it is for all original researchers, to discover that my findings have not only "rung a bell" in another soul, but have been used effectively in his own personal work. Malcolm has taken this independent research, which led to the discovery of the relationship between the color of light and the nature of consciousness, and used it to show the pathway of a Living Yoga to wholistic health.

Whoever looks at Malcolm Strutt, bursting with health, will know that the proof of all theory is in a living example. During the World Conference on Scientific Yoga in New Delhi Malcolm acted in the capacity of my right hand man, organizing a six week pilgrimage after the conference and subsequently returning to London to run Centre House and to put on thousands of classes for the London Education authority and many Yoga groups.

It was at this Conference that I introduced Malcolm to B.K.S. Iyengar whom I asked to be chairman of the Teaching and Social Action Committee of the conference of 800 yogis. Although already an outstanding practitioner, Malcolm was always ready to learn and has now brought out his own three stage course in Yoga.

He is thus the kind of student that every teacher craves for, who improves on everything he is given and who is ultimately a polished mirror of all his gurus.

PERSONAL NOTE

In writing this book I thank all those good people, known and unknown, who have influenced my spiritual growth with their wisdom, love and patience. This book is presented as a course of instruction that is a reflection of the systematic training that I have been privileged to receive and to pass on to others through my responsibilities as a Yoga teacher.

During the early years of my learning, there were three persons in particular who, to me, exemplified a spiritual master:

Paramahansa Yogananda and his teachings of the Self Realization Fellowship have been close to my heart for many years, as indeed have been the vibrations of his spiritual presence. The high standard of his devotion and teaching have acted as a firm foundation of inner stability in many an uncertain and difficult situation in my life. To him and to all those who further his work, I give my sincere thanks.

When I first saw Sri B.K.S. Iyengar giving a Hatha Yoga class I was not able to see what I could learn from such a class. Now I welcome the opportunity to work with this great man and to follow his very disciplined, yet tremendously fulfilling, love of Yoga. His inspiration and knowledge have given me so much that words are inadequate to express my gratitude. A continuing practice with greater effort is my thanks to Mr. Iyengar and also to Silva Mehta, his devoted disciple, who has guided me in his methods and training.

Christopher Hills came into my life as an interesting personality, and came to be my friend, father figure, business associate, teacher and guru. His ability to master all levels of consciousness and to reflect back to me so many sides of my nature of which I am unaware have made me wonder how such all-seeing clarity in consciousness can be attained. When he and his wife Norah were at Centre House, our Centre Community could never be complacent or without direction. Their leadership and love, both personal and impersonal, made one either grow very quickly or leave the community for some easier path. Christopher's guidance has shown me the meaning of Pure Consciousness and has led me to my guru within, who is reflecting the ONE in all, through the mirror of all life. Many of the words and concepts I now use come from Christopher and they were so entwined in my own consciousness during the six years he lived at Centre House that I am unable to distinguish them from my own words in this book. My furthering of the Centre Community is a small but grateful "thank you" to Christopher, who has given me the opportunity to share with others the principles and way of life that he initiated when he founded the Centre Community in London.

It is at this point in evolution, with the growing need for more light and universal love, that the challenge to put pen to paper and to communicate the self knowledge that has been revealed to me so far, has materialized. To help me to do this there have been the efforts of many friends in England and America. In particular, my appreciation goes to the members of University of the Trees who have undertaken to republish the original English version called *Living Yoga*. Here a special credit goes to Pamela Osborn, Susan Welker and Ary King who did the typesetting. To Evelyn Burges who checked the script and to other members of the Centre Community who have supported me in my work I am grateful. To all the many students who have encouraged me in my practice, and, of course, to the very Giver of Life who has played the song of love through all concerned with the publication of this book – many, many thanks.

To you, the reader, I wish unfoldment and growth in the best possible way, not necessarily from my words, but by your own practice and experience of *Wholistic Health and Living Yoga*.

INTRODUCTION

Before life can exist, before life can flow, before anything can grow, there has to be an urge, a desire, some driving or motivating force. The movement of cells around the body, the breathing of air into the lungs, and the transmission of nerve pulses through the spine are all brought about by the will to live, to be creative and to be conscious of that creativity, of that life and of that ONE who is willing it. When the will fades away, life fades with it; reject the desire to live and death ensues; forget the Creator and Creation becomes chaotic and confusing.

The same will that can create, can also maintain and destroy its own creation to make way for new and ever evolving expressions of itself. This is shown not only by nature around us, but also in the workings of our own body, in our own mind and in the life that we lead and experience with our consciousness. To study life in whatever shape, form or manner, all we have to do is to examine our own consciousness. Through answers to such questions as "Who or what created life? and "Why and how was life created?" can only be fully comprehended when one reaches the Supreme state of total enlightenment, we can at least look into our own life and into the workings of our own health and consciousness as it is with us here and now. With the right direction and reverence for the Life Giver, perhaps you yourself may be able actually to see who is feeding your own consciousness with arguments and questions about yourself. For who else is there but the SELF?

However big or small one cares to make it. Yet within the SELF is there not some Life Principle that is guiding it? Otherwise, how could we be where we are right now? What more can man desire than to know intimately within himself that Life Principle - call it God if you wish - and to tune to the purpose for which we have been created. To discover and to follow the direction of the Giver of Life is the message carried in every pain, every pleasure and in the

6

very experience of everything. It is also the motivation behind the writer and the student of this course.

Healthiness is a state of being well, and can be experienced on every level. Each level affects another; work more positively on a physical level and the mind becomes more concentrated. Behind a more positive action and a concentrated mind is a soul that is free with its giving. When consideration is given to right body exercise, an open mental attitude to new learning and a training in true spiritual awareness, then the whole person is acknowledged and the effect of each level is amplified to give the experience of Wholistic Health.

Whatever comes into consciousness, whether it be light signals through the eyes or sound into the ears, it is consciousness that has put it there. Close the eyes, muffle the ears, we can still see and hear the vibrations of our consciousness. Observe something as beautiful or ugly, it is our consciousness that describes it. What is more, it is ourself we describe, for is it not the state of our consciousness that determines reality, quality and relativity?

Knowing the SELF, the understanding of life and the realization of the ONE who is creating it in consciousness is the subject of this book.

Yoga means union with the source of life. Living Yoga is the finding of that union in every situation, every moment of the day. In order to know more deeply the workings of the SELF we look to a state of Pure Consciousness that is neither tainted by thought nor disturbed by any ego-centricities that limit it. Pure Consciousness is the state of consciousness for which everyone is ultimately striving. Some do it consciously, some do it unconsciously. Living yoga is a conscious search and development to increase the awareness of the Life Force in all things and to unite with it in the state of Pure Consciousness.

The aim of *Wholistic Health and Living Yoga* is to be aware of changes in consciousness. What causes them? Why do they happen? Who controls and who changes them? With this increasing awareness we look to the experience of an ever new joy in moving consciousness. A joy in living and a living in joy. However, spontaneous as it might be, joy is also created by the fulfillment of meaningful work, done with an interest and a purpose. The purpose of this course has been given above, the work which follows means a gradual awakening of an inner joy by a regular daily practice, which both develops and prepares the student of life for initiation into higher states of consciousness. This brings with it a union with the Creator and a closer harmony with Creation.

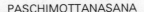

PASCHIMOTTANASANA

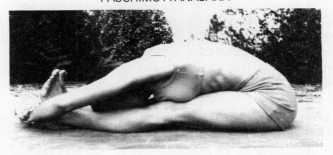

Editor's Note to the Second Edition:

In creating this expanded and highly illustrated second edition of Malcolm Strutt's book the editors wish to acknowledge the assistance readily given by Carl and Ingela Abbott and Pamela Osborn for many of the yoga posture pictures. Carl and Ingela teach Iyengar yoga in Santa Cruz and, like Malcolm, acknowledge Iyengar as today's foremost master of hatha yoga. Pamela is on the faculty at the University of the Trees where she conducts Creative Conflict sessions and teaches body awareness.

Thanks is also given to Michael Hammer, the university photographer who produced the yoga posture shots.

CONTENTS

SECTION THREE   170

OUTLINE OF THE COURSE

This book could be read simply as a book about the art of living. However, that is all it would be; a book about the art of living. To actually experience a growth in awareness and ability it is recommended that the reader fully participates in the step by step practices given in each section.

The course is given in four sections. Each is based on three fundamental laws of life. These describe the nature of consciousness and enable one to see the SELF through a study, understanding and an actualization of these laws.

It is important to follow the course at your own pace, with the right persistence and perseverance. Go too fast at anything and you will not only miss the inherent subtleties, but also burn up excessive energy. Go too slow and you may lose out on the opportunities that are here today and gone tomorrow. Become lethargic and the build-up of resistance may cause a wasting away of your energy. Likewise with persistence and perseverance; excessive "pushing" causes strain. Not enough enthusiasm, and indifference may lead one astray from the aim and intended path of action.

Guidance in recognizing the right rate of working is given in the early part of the course. For some the course may take only a few months, for others it may take years. On the other hand a deeper study and a conscious effort in practice will always bring lasting benefits. Time then is inconsequential compared to involvement and interest.

Remember that this is a way of life and can be practiced at any time. In addition to a regular morning and evening routine, there are themes which are given as a guideline for the application of consciousness to every situation in which you find yourself.

Although some Hatha Yoga postures are given in this course, they are given from the viewpoint that requires some previous posture work and body discipline. If you have not yet done this, an intensive course of practice with a good teacher or with the help of the author's Stage One and Stage Two Courses in Yoga will soon bring you up to the required standard.

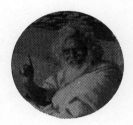

WHO IS THE TEACHER?

Your teacher is one who can reflect yourself. You will best learn from someone who has a great awareness of reality, life experience, and an ability to communicate truth to you. However, the ultimate teacher is within each and every one of us and may show himself through any person, book, or personal experience. He may also make direct contact through the faculty of the intuition. But we can only be taught if we are open and receptive. This does not mean that we take in everything that anyone says or everything that we read. Even intuition can give misleading information. Therefore we need discrimination and the willingness to test out for ourself any information that is received. An adventurous spirit, a questioning intellect, and a mind that is both ready to offer and accept challenges are therefore of definite advantage.

The age that we now live in provides more opportunities for growth and spiritual understanding than ever before. The mysteries of the occult and the secrets of the sages are not only being communicated openly, but also there are now people who do actually live the message. The West can indeed now acclaim its own yogis, gurus and teachers while the East materializes the Truths that its forefathers told and expounded.

Somewhere in all the new revolution towards evolution you may find this course a stepping stone in your own growth towards fulfillment and enlightenment. The only advice to be given here is, "Keep looking!"

A CHALLENGE TO GROW   **AN OPPORTUNITY TO SHARE**

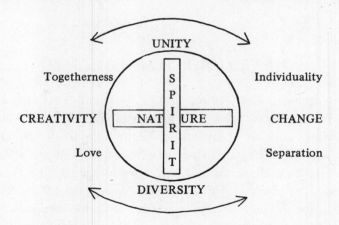

GUIDELINES FOR FOLLOWING THE COURSE

1) First participate in and experience the practical situation.
This is at the beginning of each part to be studied.

2) Read straight through the part to be studied.
Digest what you can of the text but don't worry if you find

it difficult to absorb the meaning of the words or the concepts that are presented. At this stage you are gaining an idea of a general way of looking at life and the sort of new patterns that will develop in your consciousness as the course is put into practice in your daily life. Though the actual jobs and responsibilities which you have may not change, your outlook towards them and the involvement in them could take on a completely new meaning and purpose.

3) Next read more carefully through the study material.
With the part you are studying, spend whatever time you can on seeing how it applies to you in your life. For some, after eating is a good time to digest not only food, but also the intellectual reasoning of the study material. For others a walk in the park can be a good opportunity to occupy the mind with thoughts on the text. Wherever you are, whatever you are doing, meditate and apply the theme of the part you are studying.

4) Make Time.
First thing in the morning and sometime in the evening are preferable times for the specific practical sessions that are given at the end of each part. Thirty minutes in the morning and thirty minutes in the evening is a good start. One part per month is suggested but not mandatory. It is better to take it at a pace which you can manage.

5) Start the day with an affirmation of purpose.
Upon rising look to the opportunities that the new day presents. Affirm whatever is appropriate. For example, "Today is a day for deeper study" or "Today is a day for radiating calm inner joy whatever the circumstances." Hold on to it and live it throughout the day as best you can.

6) Finish the day with a prayer of gratitude.
Reflect on the day and let go of any negative thoughts and actions. Do not judge yourself or others for mistakes. Learn

from them so they are not repeated. Pray for peace, wisdom, love and joy to shine forth from the Eternal source that is in all things and in all people.

7) Look at what your consciousness is doing.
As you meet others and go about your work, do you react? Do you mind what you are doing or how others are conducting their lives? Is there any resentment or can you be at ease in all situations? Learn how to look and listen.

8) Be honest with yourself at all times.
If you see yourself doing something that you do not want to do, find out why you are doing it. Affirm your true aim and look calmly at how you can change what may be a bad habit or conditioned action.

9) Allow change in yourself to change others.
Trying to change others without their aggreement only causes aggravation. Rather let your own efforts be the encouragement. Give advice only if you are asked. Make suggestions where applicable, but be silent when there is resistance to what you are doing. Argument creates war; creative discussion leads to positive action.

10) Be imaginative in your learning.
A tape recorder would be a useful asset for the course. To record the instructions for posture work and then to play them back while practicing the asanas means that you can concentrate on the points given at the time that they are needed. Some of the Practical Situations also require the following of commentaries which would be easier to follow from a tape recorder than from memory.

Writing things down or painting a picture of things as they are seen can be useful in learning to see oneself and in developing true SELF expression.

SECTION 1

This section explains the fundamental laws of Consciousness and starts the daily practice of experiencing them in what is common to us all right now on the physical plane — a physical body, contact with surrounding environment, and relationships with other human beings in a living situation. With these circumstances communication is important and a technique for "seeing the situation as it really is" is given.

Also,   Looking at life from the right perspective,
            Training the body for firmness and flexibility,
            Self-examination for improving discrimination.

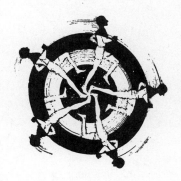

THE BODY IS A MANIFESTATION OF CONSCIOUSNESS

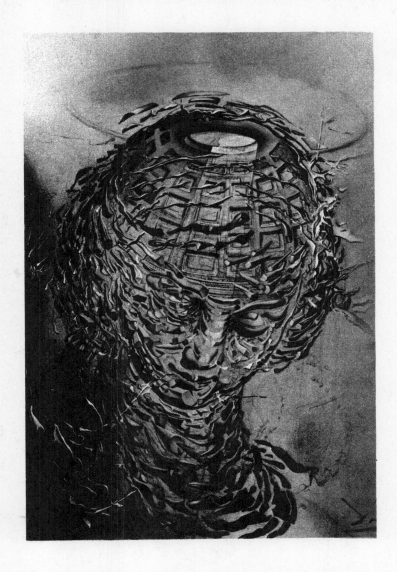

Salvador Dali, *Raphaelesque Head Exploding* (1951)

PART 1

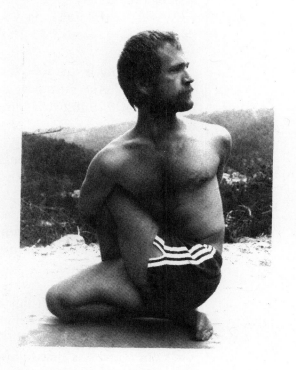

HEALTH THROUGH UNDERSTANDING CONSCIOUSNESS

PRACTICAL SITUATION -- SELF EXAMINATION

Here you are on earth with a body to move about in, a mind to drive it with and a soul to direct its course of action. For some reason or other, here you are with a yoga and health course in your hand and presumably the intention to work through it.

How and why is this so? What is your purpose in life? What meaningful attitudes and work do you see as helping you to fulfill that purpose? Is this course a part of that work?

Reflect on what went through your mind as you read the above question. Write down anything of relevance and think for the next few minutes about your philosophy of life. If you have not formed a philosophy of life, look at what it is that guides your decisions in life and what motivates your decisions in life and what motivates your actions.

When you have done this read through the study material of Part 1 and continue with the daily practice that follows it. Continue this practice throughout the week. In the weeks that follow you may find it helpful to set aside a specific time for absorbing the study material of the week. On the other hand you may find it helpful to keep the course handy and refer to it whenever you have a moment to spare. When studying it always see how it applies to you and relate it in your own terms to the life you are leading.

STUDY MATERIAL

WHAT IS CONSCIOUSNESS?

Consciousness is what we see with and what is seen. In its pure State is is the essence of life and the foundation for knowledge of the universe of experience.

Newton explained certain laws of the universe in terms of energy, showing that:

1) Energy moves from a state of rest along a uniform line of action unless interacted upon by a stronger force from another direction.

2) To every action there is an equal and opposite reaction. To which Einstein added . . .

3) Energy is neither created nor destroyed.

Though we can look at things in this impersonal and objective scientific way, we must not forget the personal subjective element of life if we are to see life and ourself both as one projection from a universal Life Force. All laws are interpreted and realized by consciousness which is individualized as a person, or life entity, and universalized as an impersonal aspect of the one all-pervading life process.

Energy cannot move without some force to move it and some awareness to guide it if it is to have meaning and purpose. If we look at Nature we see a very high degree of order. If we look at our own life we can see the same process. Who has not at some time or other wondered how on earth man came to be where he is and why he is doing what he is doing? What intelligence has guided us through the hazardous elements of circumstance and chance? One foot placed in the wrong direction or a move taken too quickly could result in our being run over by a car. A few degrees movement off course around the sun, and the earth as we now know it may no longer exist. We could be obliterated by a million and one events. Energy is somehow intelligently willed to create life with an inherent nature that relates to itself and reproduces a replication of itself that furthers the life process on many levels. In all this there is a common link – Consciousness.

The state of consciousness that sees no separation between itself and all that it experiences, is a pure state of consciousness.

Subjective experience is personal, objective analysis is impersonal. With the will that is directing   both, Consciousness is born. Yet who knows what lies behind all this in the still state of total silence from which emerges consciousness itself? (See diagram 1.1 below.)

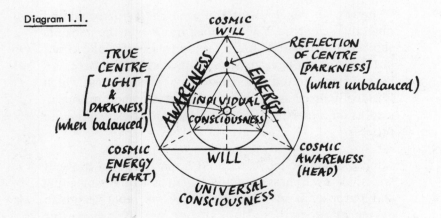

Diagram 1.1.

The balanced state of Consciousness contains the potential to create an atom or a universe, to experience both excruciating pain or ecstatic bliss. Even ignorance is only the other side of the coin of consciousness from

22

total enlightenment. In brief, everything comes out of a conscious state of being still. Let us now look at the laws of consciousness that have been chosen as a basis for this course and examine each one as it applies to a life aimed at increasing self awareness and self development towards a total SELF REALIZATION and SELF ACTUALIZATION.

LAWS OF CONSCIOUSNESS

LAW 1
CONSCIOUSNESS GOES WHEREVER WE PUT IT

Lie down, close the eyes and imagine yourself on a beautiful beach on a warm sunny day. Think about it and try to feel the warmth of the sun on your skin. Listen to the waves lapping on the shore and taste the sea air as you breath it in and out. See the blue sky and the seagulls flying overhead. Can you experience this to the extent that you become completely rejuvenated by the scene?

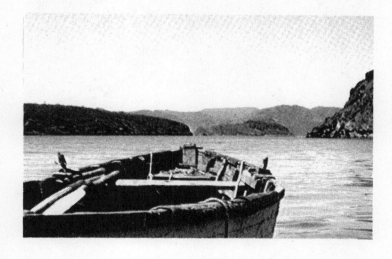

If the experience is not real enough for you and you want to experience it physically by the sea, a longing for that situation can eventually draw you to it. Whatever you ask for you can receive. This is a universal law. However, to every action there is an equal and opposite reaction so that if you want something you will receive it, but you may also receive something that you don't want. Are we not where we are now because we have put ourself here? Think about it. With concentration have we at sometime established in our consciousness an image of a body? Lo and behold here we have one. Put your hands on your face and smile --- see how the face changes. Keep smiling and it remains that way. Have you noticed the shaping of the face of someone who is always miserable? In fact the whole body droops, doesn't it? Lift the consciousness, straighten the body and wear an evenminded expression by seeing things in a balanced way. Doesn't it feel more you? Most people are hypnotized into thinking they exist in a body alone.

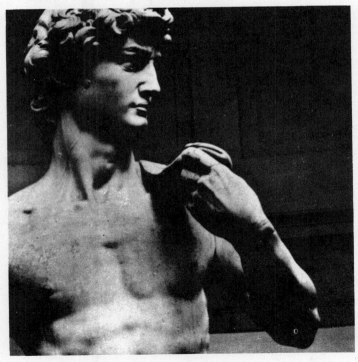

Put your consciousness on your immortal nature and see how your physical cares and worries are a result of this natural law of consciousness. Suffering is a part of life but it is only a part and when the reason for it is clear, there is a realization of its passing nature. Though at the time it may seem very real, outside of suffering and beyond it there is joy. If we can maintain the direction of our consciousness and learn to experience the joy in moving consciousness, then pain can be moved to a state of ecstasy and the situations that look black can be seen with a new light. Some create a certain kind of joy in being ill but the ultimate joy does not depend upon whether one is ill or well, it comes when one feels the presence of the God-self who knows the cause of events and has the direction and purpose to motivate right action.

The ability to move consciousness comes from an interest in it and the willingness and enthusiasm to explore it. Put your consciousness on the past by tracing thoughts backwards and you may see yourself in past incarnations, since consciousness in totality never dies. Though the body or even the mind may give way, the ONE who created the whole universe can easily create a new body and mind. Even souls are never lost completely. Put your consciousness on purifying the body, mind and soul and they will shine with the radiance of the pure consciousness from which all things are created.

Later in the course we shall learn ways of tuning to the True creative SELF. Concentrate on these practices and never look back. Like climbing a mountain – keep on towards the top. When you reach the top you will know you are there and all things will be revealed to you.

Note that when you put your consciousness in one direction there can be a strong pull from the opposite direction due to past habits. Though God helps those who help themselves, He also comes to those who are humble enough and have enough faith to receive Him. Being meek but not weak adds strength to one's bow.

In every situation life presents both an easy road and a challenge. To enjoy doing what is important and also to do willingly and cheerfully what has to be done is to do all things "as it is in Heaven." We may learn from every movement of consciousness the ways of the True SELF. From this the recognition of the ONE who is moving the whole of consciousness may come in a flash.

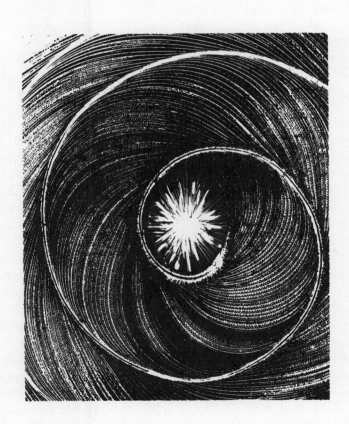

LAW 2
IN CONSCIOUSNESS WE SEE ONLY
WHAT IS OF OURSELF

Though consciousness may take on many forms and evolve through many cycles of time, in its pure state it is eternal. Neither created nor destroyed, it is re-appearing in the mirror of life and ever returning to its pure state in the still silent Center of nothingness. Since our consciousness is a projection from the still silent Center of our being it must be to this still silent center of our own consciousness that we ultimately return for the answers to life's secrets.

Yoga and meditation are a means of turning our consciousness inwards to the Center and allowing energy and awareness to express itself from that center; that is, to be quiet within and looking with an observing "I" that sees the reflection of itself in the way consciousness moves. The "I" that sees all as a reflection of itself is the God-Self. Any other self to which we attach a possessive "I" with achievements and greatness outside the abilities and qualities of others is not the "I" that is in the God-endowed state. For in that true state all beings are seen as parts of oneself and equal in potential. The ONE is in all things.

However, there is an apparent difference in all things due to this potential being manifested in different patterns. In consciousness we move energy in certain ways which form patterns and these repeat themselves until they are stopped or changed. This is the basis of habit. These patterns are called vibrations or cycles and the whole universe is built up and moves according to various combinations of these vibrations. We experience these vibrations as relative changes in our interrelated consciousness. For example, feelings are affected by the rotation of the moon around the earth. Movement of the earth around the sun is constantly affecting our creativity and receptivity through the cycles of the day and night. Vibrations from actions and

27

from thought patterns of others can also influence us to a large extent, for better or for worse. The simplest vibration is the sine wave as shown in the diagram 1.2. This is caused by a to and fro motion first in one direction, which we usually refer to as positive, and then in the other, which we refer to as negative. Whenever we project with the Will what is seen within, the positive portion of the curve is initiated and followed. Prolonging this projection eventually leads to a turning point when it is necessary to be receptive to what is happening, and this is shown by the negative part of the curve. When a person is associated with a group of others and brings forth a positive suggestion to a situation, it may happen that another member of the group reacts to it or it disturbs them somewhat. They are at this point experiencing a negative phase, and as people in the group may be "up" or "down" in their conscious state, a curve of the group consciousness may well look like that of diagram 1.2b. It is through these swings between positive and negative poles that a duality often appears.

Diagram 1.2.

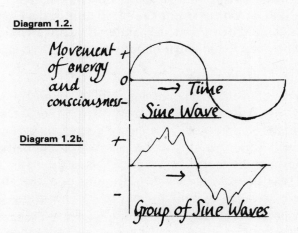

Diagram 1.2b.

If the illusion of time and space (relativity) becomes fixed by attachment to the seeming differences of negative and positive energy, then involvement without conscious evolution causes random changes in consciousness, which have no reference to the reality of life.

Man tends to forget the reason for these changes and creates his own ignorance of the reality of things by separating his consciousness into ego patterns that form the basis of selfishness. For example, if a desire for something is satisfied more than twice, a habit is formed in consciousness and after several repititons it may become apparently "natural." Although the original desire may have arisen from a real need (for instance, a certain food when hungry) several repetitions may cause it to become an apparently "natural" need, when in fact too much of any one thing can have detrimental effects. The original need is often forgotten in these cases and therein lies the cause of Ignorance. If the desire is one of self-gain or in any way a restricting of consciousness, it will bring with it an attendant pain or suffering, which is the universe's way of reflecting the state of an ego or mind-limiting consciousness. We are thereby encouraged to change to a more open and expanded state of awareness in which the consciousness flows more easily to the needs of others.

As one sees more clearly the difference between the self-limiting ego patterns and the true universal patterns, it is possible with effort, to return to the state of wholeness or at-one-ment (atonement) with the Source. Hence in the Christ-conscious state, Jesus as a person was not claiming to be God, but rather that in his consciousness he realized the Truth that in essence there is no separation between Man and God. Any seeming separation is caused by the attachment to the ego and the identification with the mind, body and senses. Purify the body and mind by discipline and the ego comes under

29

control. Purify the consciousness by nonattachment and the oneness is revealed. This non-attachment and purity was displayed by Jesus's willingness and ability to discard the body which is only a part of the total consciousness. Other great Masters have shown this ability and also the ability to rebuild the body at will.

The way in which the whole of consciousness is focused onto the screen of life by the ego can be seen in the nature of light and the way in which it is focused through a lens.

The shaping of the lens (ego) produces a prism shape at either end of the lens. This alters the direction of the light (consciousness) and introduces the seven separate colors of the spectrum: red, orange, yellow, green, blue, indigo and violet. It is interesting to note that in Hills' theory of consciousness* there are seven basic functions for the maintenance of life and seven levels of consciousness related to the different parts of the personality. These are investigated later in the course. When the lens is in the right relationship to the source and screen, the colors are clear and well defined. When the image is out of focus, the colors are muddy and exaggerated. Consciousness works exactly like this. With the ego out of place, life reflects a murky image and with the ego under control everything is in its true perspective.

Diagram 1.3

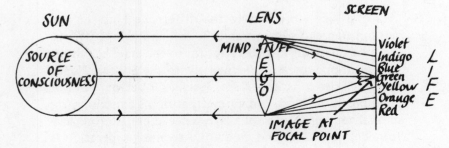

* Christopher Hills' theory of consciousness has been outlined in a book by another student, Robert Massy, in which he shares his own growth experiences by putting this theory into practice.

30

The central ray of pure light is undeviated by the lens. As with consciousness, it is that central ray of Pure Light that reflects directly the true image of the source. Containing all the colors in potential form, it serves as a reference for the focusing process. Pure consciousness is inherent in all that we see and when all parts of our consciousness are in their rightful place, our actions, thoughts, feelings, etc., are correctly focused and they reflect the radiance of the essential functions of each part in tune with the whole Being.

In everything we see there is a triune of forces. Electricity used earth as its reference for the transmission of positive and negative energy. The atom has its nucleus which keeps protons and electrons in a certain order. Even our planetary system has a sun around which planets revolve in keeping with the balancing forces of nature.

The basic ingredients of consciousness (Energy, Awareness, and Will) pervade the whole universe around us and within us alike. In fact, when we are conscious of an object it is not really outside ourself since the mind is not contained *in* anything. It is only our own self-

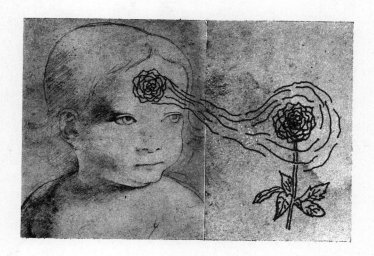

limitations, our ideas about where we stop, the boundaries of ourselves that cause separation. If we identify our self as the body all "external" objects are experienced outside. Whereas, in reality, they are experienced inside our brains, not "outside". Outside and inside become relative terms that have no reality whatsoever. The same energy is vibrating in our organ of perception --- the brain --- as it is in the object.

The only difference between any form of energy is the rate of vibration. Invisible hydrogen and oxygen, when combined in a certain way, become visible water and on cooling become solid ice. In body consciousness we see with our eyes alone and may establish, say, an iceberg floating on water surrounded by water vapor in the form of clouds. But to the initiated there is no real difference or lasting separation. A change in termperature and they can become as one vapor. Ice, water and clouds consist all of the same gases. In reality the same vapor, the same all-pervading vibration energy, the same absolute awareness and the same divine Will of God are in us all and a change of consciousness, of temperament, can bring about that realization.

Law 3
Consciousness evolves according to the interest in it and by our willingness to grow.

Consciousness builds upon consciousness. We grow when we learn how to see more clearly and with that clarity actualize what our consciousness sees to be right for the situation at hand.

Evolution comes about by the right interaction of forces of different polarity; positive/negative; male/female. The growing process is a continual sharing of energies which are produced by these dualistic forces.

32

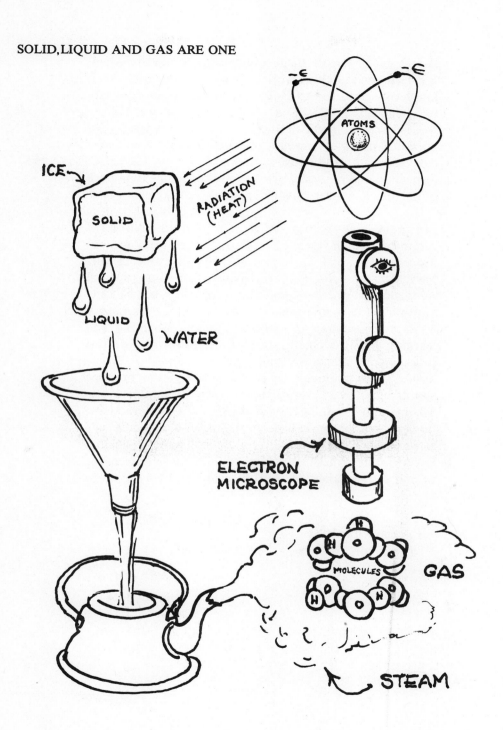

If we identify with them and become bound by them then we create delusion and cause the lower self which limits consciousness to predominate. If we can be aware, by silent observation and careful listening, we will see these forces as parts of the One Universal energy, like opposite poles of a *whole* magnet. If we expand our consciousness and direct these forces wisely, with respect to the natural way of evolution then a new state of balance and awareness will result.

Diagram 1.4 below shows the natural curve of evolution which creation follows in its ideal growth process. This is caluclated scientifically and mathematically by studying the shape, form and natural environment of plants, animals, etc. One can become aware of this evolutionary process and of the many levels of existence in oneself by experimenting and learning how to change negative tensions and doubts into positive relaxation and firm convictions of Truth. Some interactions between energies produce spontaneity and everything is seen instantaneously. Then there is no sense of time. Other interactions, however, cause separation and delusion which creates a sense of time and a sense of involution and dissolution. Greed binds consciousness whereas right self-discipline of the senses takes one into eternal time. Give time to

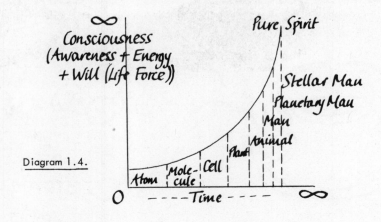

Diagram 1.4.

self development practices and time is lost for the gain of knowing the timeless qualities of the Spirit.

There are many cycles of evolution taking place in the universe. We have come through a long process of evolution without a break in the chain of reproduction, but do you remember when you were a single cell or a plant? The fact is that plants respond emotionally to the consciousness that surrounds them shows that we are all linked. Perhaps at sometime you have looked a dog or a cat in the eyes and felt the closeness of its knowing look. When atoms receive enough heightening of their energy they are ready to become a molecule. With further heightened energy (quickening of vibration) a molecule can become a cell. Molecules interact with other molecules and groups of molecules are formed. This process has developed until now we are at the stage of man. Man has the evolutionary advantage over past forms of life in that he has self awareness. With a heightening of vibration the next step for man is to live by light and increased intelligence. Those who are interested will reach that next stage. In the meantime, there is the stage of planetary man in which living in a state of supra-mental consciousness, one will no longer identify with family or country alone, but with the whole world of men.

However, man can remain man and stay where he is. Wherever we put consciousness, that is where it goes; although we may remain in a physical body, we can evolve in consciousness according to the extent of our interest and willingness to grow. There are leaders and teachers who have made that next step and draw others to themselves naturally by their light. By following their example, those others themselves become a guiding light.

We see with our consciousness, but what do we see? If we react to negative energy we have not yet evolved from the animal instinct stage. If we mind what we see we are still mind-bound. The true light of consciousness

35

lies beyond duality and the mind, and like being above in a jungle helicopter, the way is seen clearly. However, a tramp through the jungle of life may be necessary in order to confirm what is seen above by the experience below here on earth. In fact, one has not really "arrived" until one can manifest. Then, *"Thy will is done on Earth as it is in Heaven,"* and we manifest the spirituality here in the concrete world. Evolution of consciousness means an increasing ability to concentrate to a high degree and to be firm in what one sees to be the true course of action.

Evolution of consciousness also means an increasing flexibility that allows one to change and to surrender to a new course of right action as presented by the universe. Evolution means increasing awareness and actualizing it on *all* levels — physically, mentally, emotionally and in spirit.

See everything from a center of inner calm and vision will come. Look with interest and wonder at all things and evolution will take place.

Let go of old habits, religous dogma and a conditioned mind, and a new starting point will emerge.

To focus on enlightenment, what it means and how to attain it is to learn how each situation affects others. Then by seeing how everything fits in a wholesome way the self-will can become (w)holy and hence healthy.

Change increased energy, interest guides it, willingness moves it. Like the seed of a plant which has inherent in it the beauty of the flower, we too have inherent in each of us a seed that contains the light of awareness. Nurture it with yoga and meditation, give it the right environment and mix with others who are *on the same path*. That seed can then grow to unfold the inner beauty and manifestation of the True SELF.

DAILY PRACTICE FOR PART 1

THEME: OBSERVE WITHOUT JUDGING!
LISTEN WITHOUT ASSUMING!

Observe the movements of your own consciousness, your actions your thoughts, your feelings throughout the day. Don't judge them and say I should't do this or I ought to feel that. Simply observe them as they are. Do the same with the world you see around you -- people, conditions, situations, see them as they are without judgement.

LISTEN to what your consciousness is really saying. An act of, say, recklessness or an urge for excessive eating is usually a compensation for some other lack. Look at the motives for your actions and your real needs will unfold. Don't assume that what you experience is the whole truth. Listen to what your true being is trying to express. Do the same with the world around you. What appears to be a dull and windy day may be a necessity for the maintenance of life on earth. The tears of someone's emotional outburst may be an excuse to get what they want or it may be a release arising from an inner need. They may not even realize this themselves. We may express either from a pure heart or from a deceiving mind. Observe without judging, listen without assuming and the truth will be revealed in time. Be patient and be honest with yourself, but don't blame yourself or others.

MORNING ROUTINE OF YOGA

Already you may have a daily routine of yoga that is suitable for you. Alternatively you could master the routine that follows. This daily routine covers the seven basic types of posture which treat the seven main areas of the body described later in the course -- plus Savasan for the relaxation of the whole body.

Details of the mechanics of the postures are given both in LIGHT ON YOGA by Sri. B.K.S. Iyengar and in the author's three stage Course in Yoga .

In the pages which follow, we will examine the meaning and purpose of the postures and their psychological and spiritual effects on consciousness.

THE APPROACH TO YOGA POSTURES

In the practice of Hatha Yoga the body is consciously placed in a number of specific positions so that particular glands, nerve centers and sets of tissues are affected in a healthy and particular way. The manner in which postures are performed is very important. The consciousness must be calm and relaxed and focused in a non-attached yet meaningful way. The effect of this meditative state of body positioning is to bring about correct metabolic functioning of the body chemistry and a balance of the physical, nervous and emotional energies in the body. The ensuing state of peace is reflected in the mind and soul.

As the ability to both observe and to listen increases, learn how to feel yourself in the center of the body part and to know what is needed to bring it into harmony with the intended position of the whole. Consider both the whole body and the needs of its individual parts. Develop and apply firmness and flexibility so that the skin texture feels healthy.

Hatha Yoga is both a science and an art. It is the precise positioning, together with the fluid manner in which it is practiced, that produces the lasting beneficial results.

Holding a posture for a long time with ease encourages an enduring quality. Practicing a variety of postures may increase flexibility but a large number of postures should not be done at the expense of a deeper understanding of each one. Some postures such as the Dog Pose take the spine inwards towards the center and give it a movement it rarely encounters in everyday life. It is this movement and other movements, such as the spinal twist, that reach the layers of muscles close to the vertebrae which normally tend to be neglected. (See diagram 1.5).

The practice of Yoga prevents these muscles from atrophying. The decay of muscles and fibres through lack of exercise is the cause of many spinal defects. So choose the most appropriate asanas that fit your need.

Remember that we breathe all day long and that life is a series of body movements and positions. We therefore have the opportunity to observe and experience ourselves several hours each day. Use the time wisely and, when walking for example, be aware of what is happening in your body and mind. See with the soul, not with the senses.

If you sit over a typewriter all day, keep the spine straight, the chest broadened, and relax the body around the firm framework of an upright spine and shoulders pulled back.

VERTEBRAL COLUMN

Diagram 1.5.

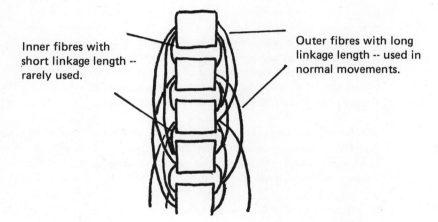

Inner fibres with short linkage length -- rarely used.

Outer fibres with long linkage length -- used in normal movements.

Consciousness itself is the means by which we gain the ability to focus on a part, become the part, and exercise that part from within. With certainty and direction you may become aware of the universal energies working through the whole body and the role that you play in the ever-evolving cycle of life.

What follows is a daily routine of asanas that will suit the needs of most people.

Concentrate on the development of the legs during this first section of the course. On this firm foundation, emphasize spinal postures in section two and inverted postures in section three.

Practice the various groups of postures daily in the order given, i.e.:

1) Standing 2) Balancing 3) Inverted 4) Backbends
5) Twists 6) Forward bends 7) Meditation 8) Lying

Practice with the following directives and questioning:

1)   Examine the state of your consciousness after each posture. Ask what are the positive effects of the posture? How can I use it for directing my consciousness? For example, you may find that standing postures uplift the consciousness, and backbends may invigorate you. Therefore if at any time you feel depressed, those postures could be appropriate. If you are not in a situation that allows you to do them, imagine yourself in the same state of consciousness as when you are doing them. You might emphasize this by simply keeping the chest and sternum lifting. allows you to do them imagine yourself in the same state of consciousness as when you are doing them. You might emphasize this by simply keeping the chest and sternum lifting.

2)   Direct the body into position from within the center of yourself. Using the energy that comes in on the inhalation, consciously move the skin in the natural direction for a perfect posture with the exhalation.

3)   Breathe smoothly and evenly throughout. If you want to make more effort,then take in more energy on the inhalation and direct it more consciously throughout the body on the exhalation, but keep the rhythm of the breathing the same and let the heartbeat adjust itself to it.

4)   Find out what the perfect shape of the posture is and what form it should take.

5)   Examine the nature of each posture and see what encourages perfect balance when doing them.

6)   At all times, maintain a consciousness that is still within, at ease with itself and open to new awareness and positive energy flow.

DAILY ROUTINE OF ASANAS

⟶ indicates a direct follow-on   ☐ indicates a repositioning for next asana.

1) STANDING POSTURES

TADASANA   **TRIKONASANA**

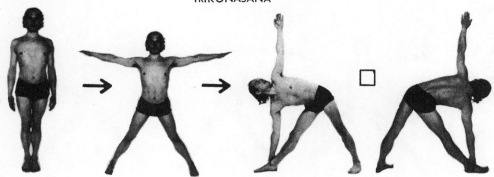

Repeat on other side   view from back

PARSVAKONASANA

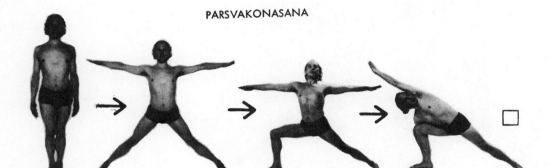

return in sequence – repeat on other side

2) BALANCING POSTURES

ARDHA CHANDRASANA

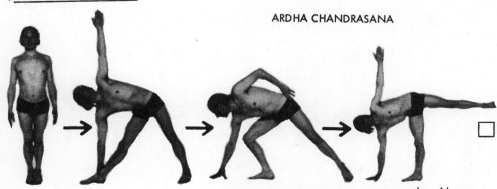

return in sequence – repeat on other side

41

VIRABHADRASANA - BALANCE

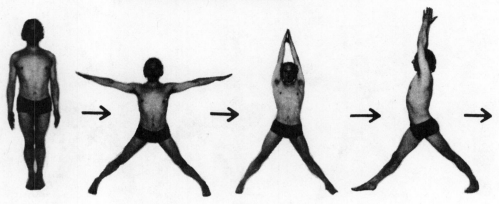

← return in sequence – repeat on other side

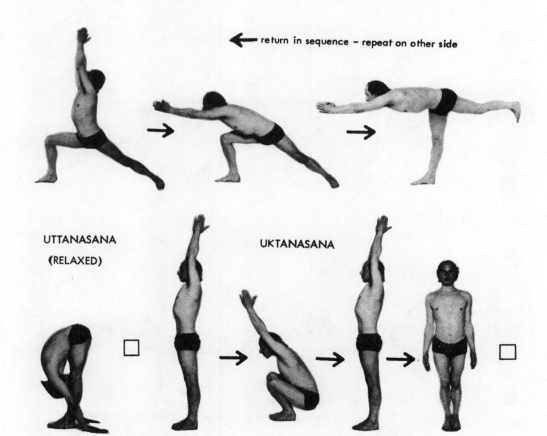

UTTANASANA
(RELAXED)

UKTANASANA

DAILY ROUTINE OF ASANAS (Continued....

3) INVERTED POSTURES

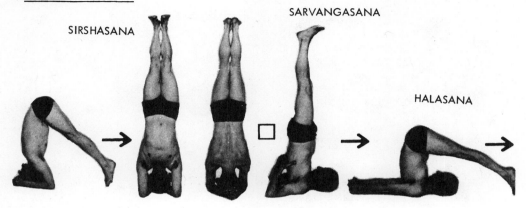

SIRSHASANA

SARVANGASANA

HALASANA

view from back

4) BACKWARD BENDS

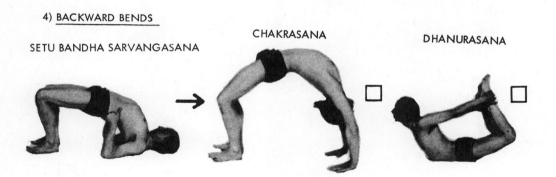

SETU BANDHA SARVANGASANA

CHAKRASANA

DHANURASANA

5) TWISTS

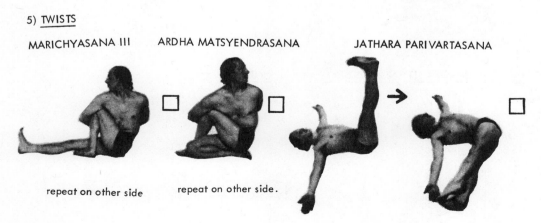

MARICHYASANA III

ARDHA MATSYENDRASANA

JATHARA PARIVARTASANA

repeat on other side

repeat on other side.

repeat on other side

6) FORWARD BENDS

ARDHA PADMA PASCHIMOTTANASANA.

repeat on other side

PASCHIMOTTANASANA

YOGA MUDRA IN VIRASANA

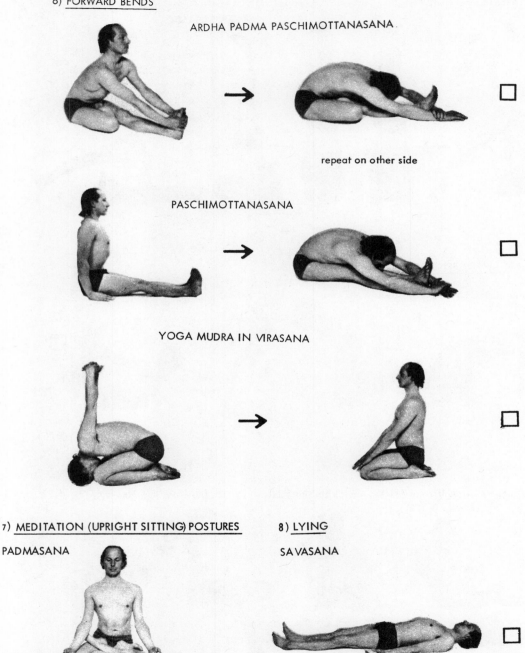

7) MEDITATION (UPRIGHT SITTING) POSTURES

PADMASANA

8) LYING

SAVASANA

PRANAYAM: HEALTH THROUGH BREATH

Lie down in a relaxed position with the body evenly palced on the ground, legs together but feet splayed evenly in a V-shape. Bring the shoulders away from the head and have the head in line with the body. Make sure that the head is not leaning too far back or too much into the chest so as to cause tension in the neck or throat. Relax completely but consciously. Close the eyes.

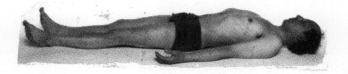

NORMAL BREATHING

1) Observe how the universe is breathing through the body. Look at it as though you were above, watching the abdomen rise with the inhalation and fall with the exhalation. Don't try to draw breath in or to fill the lungs --- merely observe what is there already. Notice the natural rhythm of the breath. Again don't interfere with it, just observe it and note it.

2) Now as the breath comes in, let it come in freely, but towards the end of the inhalation encourage it slightly. Then let it go and towards the end of the exhalation encourage the breath by gently drawing the stomach in a little.

Don't force the breath in any way; simply encourage it in its natural direction, like pushing a child on a swing. At the end of each swing just a gentle encouragement with very little effort is needed.

3) Now with the mouth closed whisper SA on the inhalation and HA on the exhalation. Listen to the breath in the throat by a slight closing of the throat, like water coming through a hose

when the opening is slightly covered. Listen to the sound of the breath. When done correctly, the mouth is kept closed, the throat relaxed, and there is an automatic SA sound on the inhalation and a HA sound on the exhalation.

4) Listen carefully to the sound of the breath and use the sound as a guide in making the breath smooth and even. Follow it very closely like you would follow a fish swimming among numerous other fish in a pond. Keep the attention on what you are following.

APPLICATION TO LIFE

Hold on to what you find to be your natural rate of breathing. Use it as a reference point and move the body either in yoga postures or in everyday work in keeping with that natural rhythm.

Listen to the sound of the breath at intervals. If it becomes jerky, hesitant or over-excited see what caused it and why. Bring it back to a steady, smooth and even inhalation to exhalation.

OBSERVE! EXPERIENCE! LOOK! LISTEN!

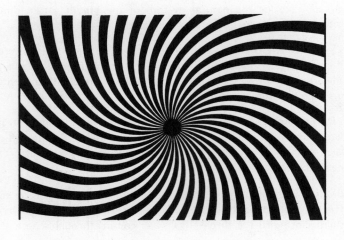

46

PART 2

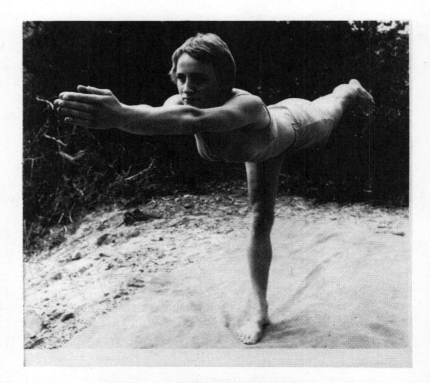

HEALTH THROUGH PSYCHO-PHYSICAL ACTION.

PRACTICAL SITUATION -- SELF ENCOUNTER

Find a friend with whom you can gaze into each others eyes. It is preferable that they are either doing this course or are into yoga, meditation or similar self-encounter work. If there is no one who understands what you are doing and who will share in this experience with you, you could, as a last resort, do it looking into a mirror. However, it is intended to be a situation with two human beings so do your best to find a true friend. It is also helpful to read and record on tape the following commentary, then to play it back before the silent encounter.

1) Sit opposite each other, relax and look at each other silently for a while. Enquire within what it is that draws you together. Is it the shape of the face? Is it the look in the eyes? Is your partner

> quiet and calm?
>
> confident or assertive?
>
> artistic or scientific?
>
> intellectual or emotional?
>
> imaginative or seemingly "down to earth"?

Is there anything in your partner that you feel is limiting the true expression? For example, is there any egocentricity, tendency to dominate, is there a shyness or a loud expression?

2) After about five minutes of this silent encountering, discuss the experience with your partner objectively and see if you can give some creative "feedback" about their positive or negative qualities that will help him or her to know the true SELF and grow.

3) Look back over the experience and see what was happening in your own consciousness. At any time did you react, feel embarrassed or imposed upon — if so, why?

48

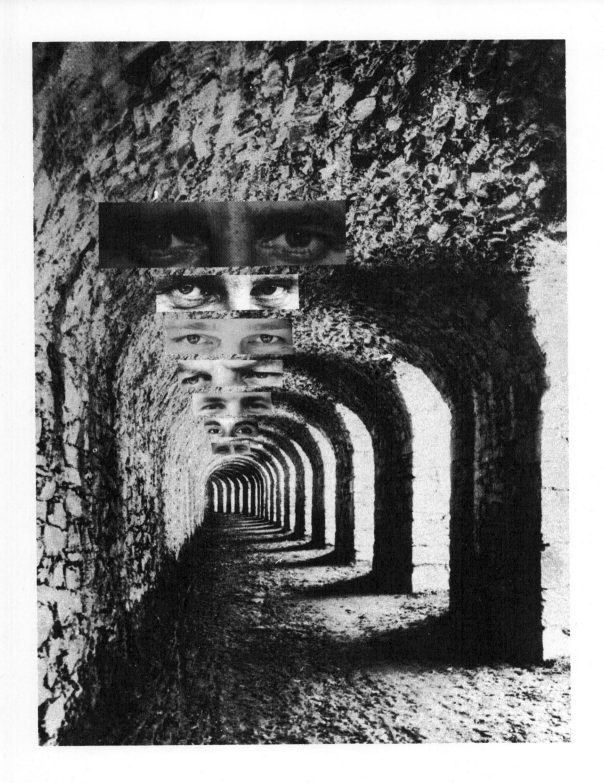

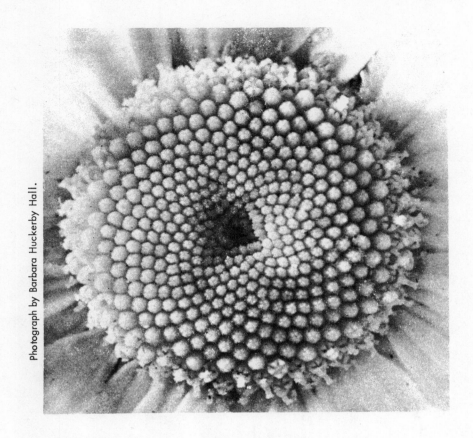

In a vision in 1957 while in his garden looking at the heart of a sunflower, Christopher Hills saw the birth of the universe in this symbol. He turned and saw it in the face of a daisy and then looked around and saw that everything in sight and all fields of energy were constructed around the same proportional principles. This symbol of the primordial atom and the spiritual sun appeared on his first book "The Kingdom of Desire" and was copyrighted in 1959. It has been used repeatedly to describe Nuclear Evolution Theory and as a visual aid to concentration of consciousness, the mandala of all mandalas.

STUDY MATERIAL

THE NATURE OF CONSCIOUSNESS

Nature itself gives a clue as to the way consciousness moves in its natural patterning. Have you ever looked into the center of a flower or at the patterns of a sawn off tree trunk? In the photograph of the daisy can you see, in the center arrangement, two spiral-like movements appear to form?

In diagram 2.1 you can see a symbol, which is based on the fundamental pattern of consciousness. The spirals of energy seen both in the flower and in the symbol can be seen throughout nature. They follow a specific mathematical law called the Fibonacci series. Exact and beautiful as they are, some invisible consciousness has created those perfect visible forms and what is more, some invisible consciousness is seeing them and is recognizing the perfection in them. The nature of their

**THE SYMBOL OF NUCLEAR EVOLUTION
DEVELOPED BY CHRISTOPHER HILLS**

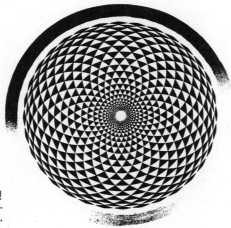

Diagram 2.1
Drawn by John Godfrey.
Photographer John Woodman.

formation reflects the nature of consciousness as it manifests.

The logarithmic curve of evolution shown on page 34 is also a natural pattern and the leaves grow out from the stalk of a plant according to this law. The human ear responds according to this law too and electricity condenses its charge between two electrodes by the same law.

Wonderful as nature is, it can also be violent and destructive. However, it invariably comes back to a state of balance. Often, what appears to be for us catastrophic, is for nature a sweeping away of the cobwebs in order to make way for a new "dawning." Applying this to consciousness, have you ever had to do some mundane task like sweeping the floor and felt just a little bit resentful at having perhaps to clean up someone else's mess? When next you feel like this, try to see how nature performs this act of sweeping away its own unwanted vegetation with the force of the wind, and how it redistributes the energy elsewhere. See how it freshens up the atmosphere for new growth. Look also at how other forces of nature, like highly developed spiritual entities, sweep up the psychic mess of those who give out resentful vibrations.

Looking at things from this broadened viewpoint you can expand your consciousness. See the difference that you bring into the act of sweeping the floor with thoughtfulness. The way in which you hold the broom and the way in which you make the strokes are all describing the state of your consciousness. This simple act of sweeping the floor can raise the level of consciousness considerably if done consciously with an interest in learning from it and with a love of sharing energy.

Nature evolves through cycles, forever returning to its origin but never to its original position in time. Since nature moves forward, not backward, every day is a new day in which the cycle of events create new opportunities and new challenges. A well known slogan that can be applied to the practice of living in the now is: *Today is the first day of the rest of your life.*

Affirming this in the morning can be a great uplift and motivating incentive to start afresh. If consciousness can be trained to see every movement in this refreshing way, can you imagine how invigorating and revitalizing life could be? Pets often show this ability to see things afresh. Give a small sign of affection and a hungry cat will purr in your lap. A playful watchdog can become a ferocious animal at the sign of an intruder. Nature changes according to the situation in order to bring about a balance and order. Change without meaning can be dangerous. From a state of balance (inner calm) evolution can progress with ease.

It is this ability to become still and balanced that prepares one for the privilege of receiving more awareness. Moving consciousness with this clarity and humility makes for a smooth journey to enlightenment. Move without this ease and the movement creates more disease. Struggle into a yoga posture or tense in it and the posture will reflect that tension. What is more, *consciousness goes where we put it.* Repeat the performance and a habit is started. Also, *consciousness builds on consciousness.* A repeated bad habit builds an unsteady foundation for further development. On the other hand, a good habit repeated gives a firm foundation and opens up the way for more creativity. Hence, it is important to start a posture or other movement of consciousness in the right way: with concentration balanced by an inner calm.

A balance and inner calm is also developed by repeated actions that encourage this state. The breathing exercises given in this book and the attitude of looking and listening as described in Part One assist this process.

BALANCE OF YIN AND YANG

Energy vibrates and moves in cycles. The Yin (ingoing energy) and the Yang (outward expression) are interrelated and are shown balanced in the symbol of diagram 2.2. This Yin/Yang symbol depicts the nature of consciousness. Even though one may have inner calm, too much of a tendency in a certain direction will eventually lead to a conflict situation between the inner calm and outward activity, if there is not a balance with physical relaxation and inward introspection. The result could be a heart attack or mental disturbance.

Since nature always tends towards balance, eventually everything becomes its opposite, and SELF may see its SELF in all things. Therefore, to do wrong to someone is to set the wheels in motion whereby the situation is reversed and oneself is being wrongly treated. This is the law of Karma - action and reaction (Law of Consciousness No. 2).

Knowing how to combine opposites is a skill perfected by the enlightened person. To be actively calm and to be calmly active in tune with one's true nature is to be at ease in a blanced state.

Diagram 2.2.

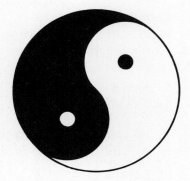

54

Activity and Passivity are two of the three main forces of our nature (and therefore of consciousness) that we need to know how to balance. The third force is a neutralizing and controlling one.

Stand with the feet apart as in Trikonasana and experience moving the body over towards the left leg. Notice how that left leg becomes active and the right one passive. Notice that the force at the pelvis is neutral and yet it contains the potential for both activating and passifying elements.

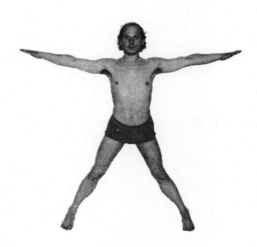

Press the right foot harder on the ground without moving the body. Notice how there appears to be more weight on the right leg. Your consciousness has created that activity in the right leg and also the feeling of more weight, has it not? In other words, consciousness when not properly balanced creates the illusion of weight. Contrary to this see how "light" you become when you are balanced and keep the consciousness lifted.

THE THREE GUNAS

In yoga philosophy the forces of activity, passivity and neutrality are called Raja Guna, Tama Guna and Sattwa Guna respectively. When one can see all three at work and balance them ,then one is in the Centre of Consciousness. In the Centre of Consciousness there is perfect balance and one is at rest. (See diagram 2.3.).

Diagram 2.3.

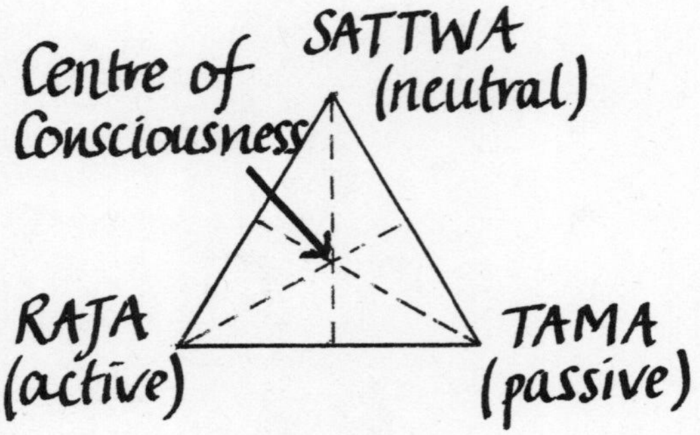

The "Triune of Natural forces" (the three Gunas) can be seen throughout nature. In growth and movement the active element is easily seen, but there is also a passive element and a controlling element affecting the growth. In the body, while one part is active another part is passive, the controlling force is the balancing force of the discriminating "I" that identifies with and recognizes what is in balance and what is out of balance. The observing "I" that sees and experiences all three forces, ever changing in their relative movements around the whole body, is the centred SELF.

The nature of consciousness is to focus and reflect the Centered Self an every-changing interaction of the three Gunas. Although the reflection displays the Self, moving in the energy patterns caused by the three Gunas, the reflection is not permanent. Hence life is showing an image of the SELF which is both illusory, in the sense that it is ever changing, and real in the sense that it can be experienced and recognized as emanating from a permanent but unseen CENTER within one's SELF. How is this so? Well, how does one see one's own face? We may know that something is there by contacting it or experiencing it with another part of our being. As long as we can be still within we can see all things emanating from that still center of pure existence. By looking at a reflecting surface through the experience of the senses we see the expression of consciousness from that still center, and see the effects of physical movements, inner emotions and psychic contact with the vibrations of the environment. Life is a mirror. To look at the cause and nature of life's movements is to look at the reflection of the causations and natural patterns of energy that move our own consciousness.

Though life moves on and nature's setting may change, the ONE who is in the Center is the Eternal viewer of the cosmic drama called Life. So the question to ask oneself is "Where do I stand in all this?" "Who am I?" "Am I the effect of causation, the body, mind, etc., or am I in the center, at one with the causative force of creation?" "What do I see when I look into my consciousness?" "What do I sense when I feel for my own essence?"

Observing this inward movement of CONSCIOUSNESS, one may see the subtleties of an "I" that is sensitive to both the positive and the negative forces in oneself. Using a will that is centered in Truth one may stretch and expand the consciousness to control a wider swing of these positive/negative, active/passive energies.

DAILY PRACTICE FOR PART 2

THEME: STRETCH BUT DON'T STRAIN!
RELAX BUT DON'T COLLAPSE!
BE CENTERED!

In the moving of consciousness it is necessary to maintain a balance of the three Gunas. The tree of life is reflected in the tree of knowledge and what is known inwardly to be the center of consciousness - at rest and at peace with itself - can be lived when balance is maintained through every action. A steady body, even-mindedness and a calm radiance reflect the true SELF. Imbalance and conflict relfect dis-ease and it is then not easy for conscious-ness to see its true SELF.

Too much Raja Guna and activity turns into aggression.
Too much Tama Guna and passivity turns into lethargy.
Too much Sattwa Guna and neutrality turns into indifference.

What is the state of your consciousness right now? A state of calm, non-attached, but interested involvement is the centered state.

POSTURE PRACTICE

Practice postures with the following questions and directives:

1)   What is each posture saying?
What does a triangle mean in terms of experience? To experience the triangle pose fully is to understand the triangle of natural forces explained in the study material.

Experiment to see the effects of doing postures in an active, passive and neutral way. Note the effects upon the body and the difference in the texture of the skin when each one is exaggerated.

What does each part of the body and each posture mean on another level? For example, besides being a valve for the blood flow around the body, the effect or role of the heart is to revitalize the body. But what in life is the heart of anything? What does bending over backwards for someone mean in life? Can a backbend help to do this?

2)   Fit the posture to the breathing!

Practice keeping the breath at a steady rate and fit the postures to the normal cycle of breathing. Put consciousness into aiming for the perfect posture and follow through that aim by. . . . . . .

a) Observing on the inhalation - see what needs to be done to place the body in the perfect posture.

b) Stretching on the exhalation - surrender to the perfect posture, directing the body into position from within.

c) Stilling the consciousness at the end of the exhalation - make any slight necessary adjustments. Keep the consciousness directed on the perfect posture and wait for the next breath to come in.

Repeat these three steps maintaining a direction towards the perfect posture and work towards it in a calm quiet manner stretching only on the exhalation. See what you are doing and how you are doing it. See what limits movement and look for ways to unlimit it, working within your own capacity. Look for the cause of any limitation and re-program that part of your consciousness in the right direction. For example: when pain is experienced in stretching, it may be from either an unused muscle being made to work - that's O.K! or it may be from an over--tensing of a weak part - that's not O.K. When the consciousness is more concerned with the pain than on aiming for the perfect posture, then either change to a variation of the posture (a change is often as good as a rest) or come out of the posture and relax.

Since consciousness goes where we put it, putting it on the pain only increases the pain just as sympathy does not really help someone in trouble. A non-attached but concerning look for an improvement of a situation from a calm perspective is required for a creative solution. It is by concentrating in a relaxed way that the real situation can be seen.

Relaxing is not lapsing into a sleepy state. True relaxation is a conscious state in which energy is equally dispersed. Concentrating in a relaxed way and relaxing in a concentrated way from a centered state of consicousness is meditation (literal meaning - wisdom action).

Let every posture be a meditation. Learn how to STRETCH IN A RELAXED WAY and TO MOVE CONSCIOUSNESS WITH EASE.

3) Extend fully in all postures.

When stretching the arms, extend beyond the fingertips. Follow the stretch back to its origin and when stretching forward with the arms in, for example, a forward bend or twist, stretch not only the arms, but also the body from the pelvis to beyond the fingertips. Feel the skin moving from your inner direction and make every square centimeter of skin on the body alive and vitalized. Note the natural movement of energy around the body. For example in standing postures let positive energy (and confidence) rise up the front of the body while negative energy (and fear) descend down the back of the body.

Note how you feel when the front of the body droops in the standing position - unnatural, isn't it? Following the natural direction   lift upwards and broaden across the front so that the consciousness too becomes lifted and ready to face the challenges of life.

The photographs which follow show the direction of some of the skin movements in various standing postures.

As a general guide to this type of posture, keep an inner relaxation with an outer firmness. Aim for straight lines in the basic shape of the posture and turn the skin of the body in the direction indicated by the arrows on the photographs.

TADASANA   TRIKONASANA

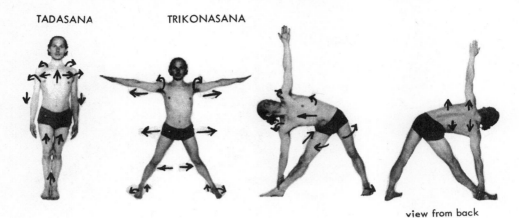

view from back

REVERSE TRIKONASANA

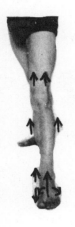

The photo of the leg in standing postures
shows the extension of the inner edge
of the leg and the firmness in the
positioning of the foot, such that the
outer edge is flat on the ground.

Note the lift up the front of the leg and
of the top corners of the knees equally
at either side of the centre line of the
leg.

The back of the legs in standing postures
needs to be broadened so that the knees
go well into their sockets and the
skin expands equally from the centre of
the legs to the outer edges of them.

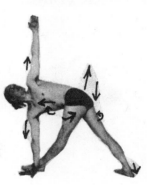

PARSVAKONASANA   REVERSE PARSVAKONASANA

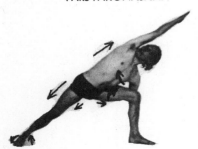

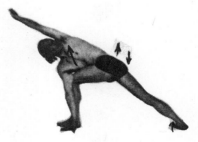

VIRABHADRASANA

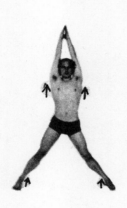 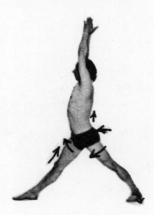 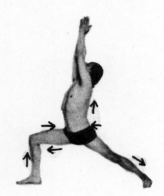

ARDHA CHANDRASANA

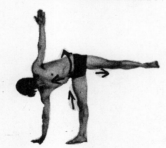

VIRABHADRASANA – BALANCE

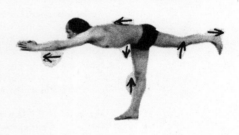

UTTANASANA

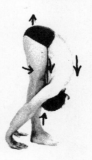

UKTANASANA

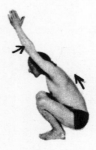

PRANAYAM: HEALTH THROUGH BREATH

Lie down and breathe as in Part 1. Continue as follows:

1)   Note how throat breathing gives control over physical energy and increases it. Guide the breath into the lungs in an increasing manner as in Part 1, and notice on the inhalation the tendency of the abdomen to rise, then the rib cage to expand sideways and then the sternum to lift towards the chin. On the exhalation, let the breath flow out naturally, finally taking in the stomach just slightly.

2)   Now put all the attention in the nostrils and guide the breath up the center of the nostrils, close to the septum. Repeat for a few minutes and note the coolness on the inhalation and the warmth on the exhalation. Don't let the nostrils flare out. Refine the breathing.

3)   Note the freshness in the head and the clarity of the mind. Note the length of the breath.

4)   Combine and balance nostril with throat breathing.

APPLICATION TO LIFE

The ability to expand one's consciousness and to see the true SELF follows the same pattern as learning to do correct postures. The ways you find for mastering a posture apply to mastering the situations in life: observe, experience, stand firm and surrender to what has to be done. Master a posture and it will reflect in another area of life. Similarly, bad posture and poor breathing will reflect in everyday work. Apply the laws of consciousness and the methods given above without letting words like *Hatha Yoga, Housework or Career* separate one from the other. Yoga is a way of life - learning how to live life to the full. Let every moment be a meditation - guided by wisdom. Let every move-ment be Yoga - fulfillment in action.

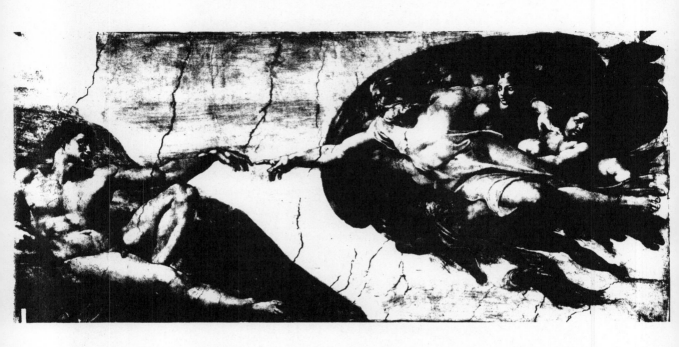

MICHELANGELO. *The Creation of Adam,*
detail of the Sistine Ceiling. 1508–12

PART 3

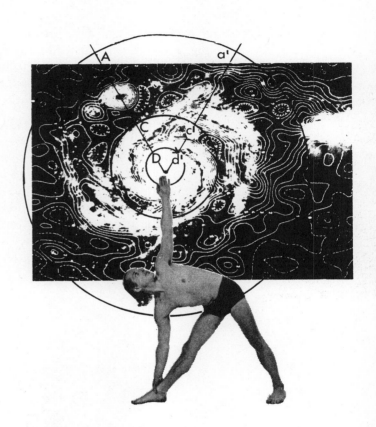

MIND-BODY
HARMONY

PRACTICAL SITUATION – SELF REFLECTION

Find a friend as you did in Part 2 for this is a similar situation. If you cannot find a friend you can in fact use a mirror. Continue reading below or record beforehand.

Face each other and look into the eyes as if you were looking into a mirror. Instead of analysing as you did in Part 2, let the eyes speak to you and receive all they have to say in a calm, relaxed manner. Remember you are looking at yourself. (Two minutes silence.)

Silently ask yourself *"How did that face I am looking at come to be?"* (Pause) *"Who is the one behind this face?"* (Pause) *"What will it become in the future?"* (Pause) *"Who will be the one behind it then?"*

Relax and discuss with your friend what you both saw reflected in the situation. If you were alone and used a mirror, contemplate what you saw.

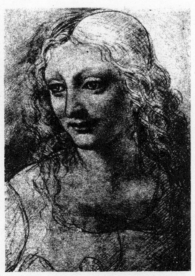

Leonardo – Windsor, Royal Collection

STUDY MATERIAL
THE FUNCTIONS OF CONSCIOUSNESS

In Part 1 we examined the fundamental laws of consciousness and in Part 2 we looked at how and why the nature of our consciousness expresses these laws of the life principle. We now come to the functions which make it possible for that expression to take place in the way that we experience it.

Life exists by virtue of forces of attraction and repulsion. Life evolves and involves itself according to the way those attractions and repulsions interact. The interaction of energies is happening on all levels and right now there are millions of cells in our bodies reproducing themselves, working together and living together. Some are separating and some are waging war against each other. Others are harmonizing and creating new patterns of energy in order that the whole body may evolve to a new level when the time is right. The patterning is important, and the functions of life create the right patterns through the right use of what has been formed already.

If we rightly use the energies and intelligence that we have already, then that right-use-ness (righteousness) is reflected in our life and we are ready to receive the next step for our evolution. There are stages of readiness.

When a person says "I can't" that is what happens. By saying "I can't " one imposes a limitation and a rationalization, for it really means "I won't." When "I can't" is changed to "How can I?" a person is then open for receiving information. When that person hears the information but does not listen, that "How can I?" simply means "I wish I could." When that wish becomes a real desire to learn, "How can I?" changes to a need and the question becomes "God, will you show me how I can?" The person then becomes a student of life ready to receive instruction in whatever form it may come, possibly through either a person, or a book or a situation. But even here a readiness for learning is not necessarily reached. What the student may be saying, consciously or unconsciously, is "Give me a demonstration and tell me how I could do it, and I will then decide whether or not I will do it." The true state of readiness comes when "Seeing" and "Being willing" come together in attentive action.

The raw materials of consciousness are energy, intelligence, awareness and will. The will cements together the mixture of awareness and energy to form a foundation for further development. In consciousness we experience this cementing process as an interaction between the male (creative) and female (receptive) energies. The manner of the relationship between these aspects determines the nature of the child that is born. Here the child can refer to an image, an idea, a concept, a feeling, a discriminating process, a social standard or a physical shape.

In life the normal family situation reflects the truth of the union of the basic principles of consciousness and their nature. When male and female energies are balanced without a dominance of any one person's character, then the marriage is stable and the child is a confirmation of this state of affairs. The child can then develop to produce a new family situation with new ideas and a pattern of life that has inherent in it this childhood stability. The more in tune the parents are with life, the stronger will be the opportunity for further growth. In a group situation an equal sharing of responsibility and creativity by its members brings about a maturing of ideas, aims and new standards in group consciousness.

There is an order to things, which is evidenced by life in its evolution throughout existence. There are certain energies that have come from the true union of the

68

primeval creative and receptive forces. These energies form the basis for further development of life and provide a function for thinking, sensing, imagining, etc., which in turn produce stable physical organisms that the children of sensation, thought and imagination have produced.

When the state of consciousness is reached in which, at that moment in time, nothing else in the world matters except to do this thing because it has to be done and because no other move can take place until this thing is mastered, then the question is a silence, and there is simply a looking and a listening. Any instruction and teaching that is given is then a blessing, from which comes the fulfillment of the need and the fruits will bear witness to the nature of that need. If it is a real need others will benefit from the fulfillment. If it is a selfish want rather than a real need the motivation will be shown in the effect of the outcome.

When the initial question is a sincere "What is truly the most important thing for me to be doing in my life at this moment?", can'ts, won'ts, woulds and shoulds no longer exist in the vocabulary and limitations start to fall away. What life brings is the need at that time, but not necessarily for all times. The same need at another time may bring a different kind of message for fulfillment. As we are reminded in Ecclesiastes "To everything there is a season, and a time to every purpose under heaven." (Ch. 3, v. 1).

If we look at the functions of life as consciousness, evolving patterns will be reflected by the wholeness and purity of consciousness. The Zodiac, the I-Ching, the patterns of nature and our own human body are all maps of consciousness that reflect basic energies and drives that make it possible for consciousness to see itself. Life in the human body has evolved over millions of years, but as far back as the basic one-celled entity, the amoeba, and probably even further back, there can be seen a series of functions which create a life pattern. These functions are:

1) *A reproductive system that furthers life* and establishes contact on the physical plane.

2) *Mobility.* An irritability and conductivity which encourage a contact with the environment to take place, and the elimination of unwanted energy.

3) *A digestive system* that takes in food energy, and redistributes from it what is necessary for the growth of the organism.

4) *A vitalizing (circulatory) process.* This is the heart of the organism that gives the will to live by virtue of its magnetizing or attracting force.

5) *A metabolic (respiratory) controlling mechanism* that keeps a balance of the above four functions.

6) *Contractability.* A nervous system gives the cell the ability to go within itself. A sort of instinctive or intuitive knowing element feeds information to all parts of the cell and controls its automatic responses.

7) *Adaptability.* A nervous system which enables the cell to survive in changing environmental conditions. This is like a creative image-making faculty that forms new patterns for future cells.

The diagram 3.1. shows the human body with similar main areas of consciousness and their corresponding body parts associated with the different types of energy, and is a result of original research by Christopher Hills. In his book *Nuclear Evolution: Discovery of the Rainbow Body,* Christopher Hills takes the reader deeper into his multi-leveled self.

Diagram 3.1.

FUNCTION	ASSOCIATED AREA OF SPINAL COLUMN	ASSOCIATED GLAND	ASSOCIATED ORGAN
Adaptability/ Parasympathetic Nervous System	Cerebrum	Pineal	Upper Brain (Ear Lobes)
Contractability/ Sympathetic Nervous System	Cerebellum	Pituitary	Lower Brain Hypothalamus
Metabolism/ Respiration	Cervical	Thyroid	Lungs
Vitality/ Circulation	Dorsal	Thymus	Heart
Digestion/ Skeleton	Lumbar	Pancreas	Liver
Mobility/ Elimination	Sacral	Adrenals	Kidneys
Reproduction/ Sensation	Coccyx	Gonads	Reproductive Organ

71

Each area has a purpose and function. For example, the purpose of the legs is to express the inner consciousness more fully by contact with the physical plane. Their function is to support and give flexible movement to the body. This provides the guideline as to what to look for in the development of the legs. An even spreading of the feet upon the ground gives a stable base to the supporting legs. The best support comes when the legs are straight and firm. Movement comes best when joints at hips, knees and ankles are flexible. Note that the knee joints do not turn left and right, but move forwards and backwards. Knees that turn inwards or outwards do so because of a malalignment in the pelvic joints or ankles.

Each area can be looked at in this way. Ask yourself, "What is the purpose and function of this area?" "How can that purpose and function be effectively fulfilled?" The physical centers associated with the seven basic functions are given above. Further explanation of their deeper aspects will be given later.

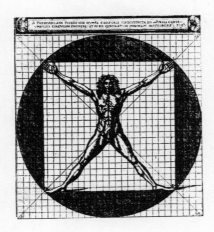

Proportion is another guideline as to the state of perfection of the consciousness. When the distance from fingertip to fingertip with the arms outstretched is equal to the distance from head to toes then spirit balances nature and actions balance aspiration-come-manifestation.

Proportions such as length of spine to length of leg are also important for physical and mental balance. The postures of Hatha Yoga bring about a perfect proportioning of the body structure. Postures like Paschimottasana help to stretch the spine. Standing postures straighten the legs. With the correct proportions and alignment there is a maximum efficiency and a perfect patterning for reflecting the true SELF.

The right relationship to others in life also makes for perfect patterning. Place total dependence upon others and one is a slave and a puppet. Total independence leads to isolation and separation. An intelligent sharing with an imaginative spirit meeting the real need of the moment, is creative. Too much attending to the growth of others without the corresponding individual growth leads to a lack of self-knowledge. Too much individual growth without the corresponding sharing of it leads to a lack in understanding. A balance in all things is the safe way to grow. Make a deep study in one field of research but be open to the research of others and their fields of study. All are related to the source of consciousness.

Your approach to any task in life will be reflected in others. An aggressive nature draws a negative reaction. This can be seen in postures as well as in relationships and situations. Meet others with a calm disposition, and the positioning of the body will be calm. Become agitated with those who don't do things as you want them to, and the breathing will become agitated. Relate to the body like relating to a person and an understanding of the actions and reactions of others will unfold.

Breathe in the way you would like life to flow and an understanding of the nature of others will increase.

Nature allows freedom but within a certain framework. Diversity is a gift of life. The refining of it and the sacrifice of it to a unity on a higher level is the function of that framework. The framework of the body and its parts provides a means for refining the consciousness that lives in it. Refining means exercising and working out bad habits that cause a malfunctioning. When this is realized the process can be refreshing --- or frightening. The choice is up to the individual --- the ONE who is undivided from the SELF that sees all as itself, moves according to a synthesis of the motivating energy and the true need.

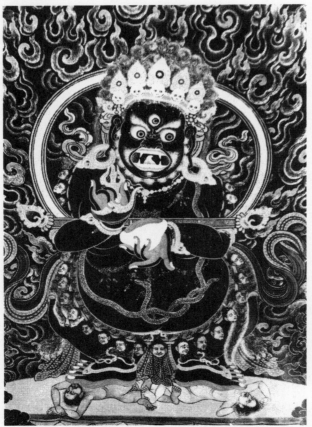

The Tibetan God, Mahakala, represents the true self's ruthlessness in cutting through the ego. He is often shown as a giant form crushing small tortured human egos under his feet.

74

DAILY PRACTICE FOR PART 3

THEME: WHAT IS ME?
*   WHAT IS NOT ME?*
*   WHAT IS THE TRUE REALITY?*

"Ask and it shall be given you; seek and ye shall find; knock and it shall be opened unto you." (Mathew, Ch. 7, v. 7.)

This message of the Bible echoes the love of the universe. Though we have free choice, we must also face our destiny resulting from the choices we make and therefore it is important to ask ourselves what we really want of life and even more important, what does life need from us?

Life is a gift and consciousness can make that gift wholesome or degraded. By bringing order out of chaos, a universal need is being fulfilled. By releasing what is no longer valid, a deeper Truth is allowed to unfold and to manifest itself. Understanding the basic functions of life and its natural patterns will give a direction in life. Participating in bringing about that natural patterning and functioning will help one to realize the reality of things. The realization of Reality brings one closer to God, but this closeness is a personal affair and cannot be discussed, any more than a kiss between lovers can be talked about. In doing so the purity and perfection of its essence is somehow lost.

POSTURE PRACTICE

If we look at the postures of Hatha Yoga from the point of view of the purpose and function of each part of the body then the direction of energy flow in a posture becomes clear. For example:

The LEGS AND PELVIC AREA govern physical movement and our relationship with the earth environment. Straightness in the legs comes with a lift up the front, a stretch on the inner and a broadening at the back of them. Lifting the ankles and top corners of the knees uplifts the physical energy from the earth. Stretching on the inner edges of the legs steadies oneself and a broadening of them across the back keeps one in touch with the world. The placing of the feet on the ground establishes a firm contact with the earth. When standing, the triangle made by the center of the heel at the apex and the ball of the foot as a base can act as a guideline when walking. Placing the toes down first you will notice a sort of cautious movement, almost like walking on thin ice. Placing the heel down hard creates a rather domineering attitude. So the skill in walking becomes one of placing first the heel, then the ball of the foot in a light but definite manner. The knees are the center or heart of the legs so keep them lifted and pointing in the direction of movement. Keeping the back of the knees broadened helps to provide a secure socket in which the knees can rest. The knees are very delicate and need to be well looked after. Muscles at the back of the legs are quite elastic in nature and can often be stretched more than we think.

The PELVIC AREA affects the direction of the legs so a looseness in this area helps the flexibility of the legs. In the standing postures the legs and pelvic area are developed in a dynamic manner. However, opening up the groins and stretching the legs cannot be truly effective unless there is also a relaxing of any tensions that are already present.

The TRUNK (base of spine to neck) governs the mind energies and our attitude towards others. A straight spine creates a strong mind. A flexible one gives flexibility in action and adaptability to situations in life. The body links the psychic energies of the head to the physical movement of the legs on the earth plane. It also raises the physical energies to the awareness of the spirit through action. The spine carries to and from the brain subtle currents of life force which give energy and alertness to it. A bent spine causes a restriction of these energies so that a continually bent spine results in a dullness of the brain and old age creeps in.

Forward bends and twists help to elongate and massage the spinal tissues and vertebrae. This "heightens" the intellect. The broadening of the chest in twists broadens the mind. At the same time the flexing action of the heart area flexes the feelings of the mind and gives more capabilities for emotional expression and action through the arms, which determine how much of "life" we embrace.

The central line through the body is the Center of Consciousness. Taking the spine inwards towards this center takes the mind inwards. Taking the shoulders back relates the action of the arms to the inner being. With the skin of the arms turning outwards there is an openness to receive from and give to the universe. However, be careful that the chest is not thrown out: this shows vanity. Rather than this, lift the chest --- that shows maturity. Better still, let the body rest evenly around a straight vertical spine and an extended horizontal collarbone. Then there is purity.

The HEAD governs the sending of psychic currents as nerve pulses through the spine to all parts of the body. It houses the brain which relates to the central spiritual reservoir for feeding the mental and physical processes with the essential motivating stimuli.

The NECK AND THROAT govern what we swallow in more ways than eating food. A person with a stiff neck is conservative in values whereas a loose neck indicates an acceptance of changing authority. Too loose, however, and there can be an idolized swooning effect towards the authority of others.

If the CHIN is lifted too high you appear to be a snob. Drop it too much and you undermine yourself. Keep the head lifting from the crown for correct posture and the underneath of the chin parallel to the ground for level-headed consciousness.

The MOUTH allows us a form of expression. Lips that are horizontal and even create an even-minded expression. The EYES govern what we see or do not see. Always looking down to the earth is no better or worse than constantly looking up to heaven and being oblivious of what is here on earth. The centered person faces both heaven and earth with equanimity. Look more through one eye and the energy is drawn to that side of the body, emphasizing either the male aspects (right) or female aspects (left). Penetrating evenly through both eyes, a balance is maintained. Broaden the BROW for a spreading of ideas into the world and lift it for a more refined level of thinking.

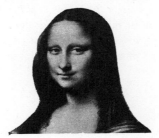

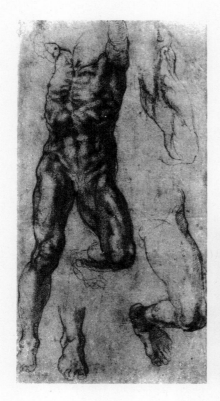
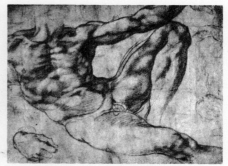

DIRECTIONS

Feel the three major sections of the body (head, trunk and legs) detailed above. Relate to each of these parts in the postures and also to the body as a whole. Note the effects of each one relative to the other. For example, when the head goes towards the feet, the soul moves towards the earth. In Paschimottanasana this creates a mothering or nurturing effect upon the body as well as directing life force to certain organs of the body. Look for the interrelationship of physical parts, mental attitudes and spiritual states in each posture.

78

EXAMPLES OF SKIN MOVEMENTS IN INVERTED AND VARIOUS OTHER POSTURES.

SIRSHASANA

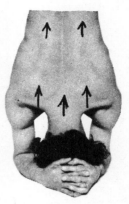

SARVANGASANA

HALASANA

SETU BANDHA SARVANGASANA

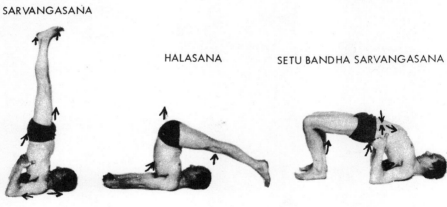

CHAKRASANA

DHANURASANA

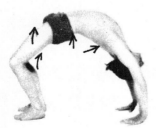
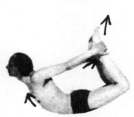

ARDO MUKHA SVANASANA   MARICHYASANA III   ARDHA MATSYENDRASANA

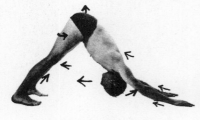 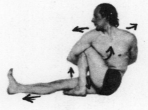 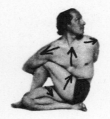

JATHARA PARIVARTASANA   ARDHA PADMA PASCHIMOTTANASANA

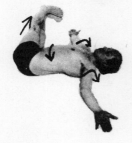 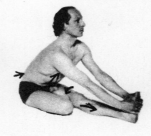 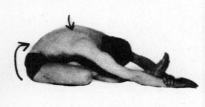

PASCHIMOTTANASANA   YOGA MUDRA FROM VIRASANA

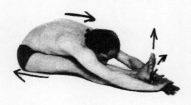 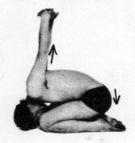

PADMASANA

SAVASANA

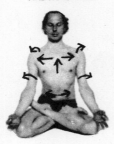 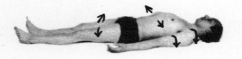

PRANAYAM: HEALTH THROUGH BREATH

Lie down and breathe as in Part 2. Note the rhythm of the breath and let it continue to flow naturally and uninterruptedly.

Continue as follows:

1) Observe the breath coming in through the nostrils, through the throat and into the lungs. Observe it going out through the throat and through the nostrils.

2) Note the part of consciousness that is observing and the part of consciousness that is breathing. Note any variations from a smooth even flow of the inhalation and exhalation.

3) Now follow the breath closely and experience the cool refreshing sensation on the inhalation and the warm comforting feeling on the exhalation. Use this experience to gradually make the breath more smooth and even.

4) Keep the attention focussed. Observe the effect, experience the cause. Differentiate what is a sensation, which gives only a feeling of satisfaction, and what is creating a life flow of pure essence. Let your consciousness be in the SELF that is pure.

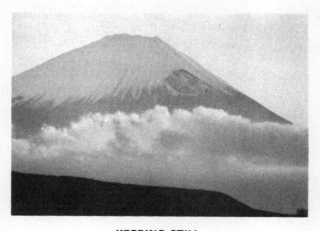

KEEPING STILL

81

APPLICATION TO LIFE

As stated earlier, relating to the different parts of the body is just like relating to people, animals, plants, work or play. With the right relationship and nourishment we encourage in ourself a certain "response - ability" and receptivity to the real needs of the undiscovered parts of ourself. Growth in terms of increased intelligence, understanding, vitality and creativity are the results of good relating. A healthy relationship is one in which the effects of actions, thoughts and feelings of each part upon the whole is considered, without allowing reactions and emotions to disturb the inner harmony. Order comes out of this kind of relationship, the whole benefits from it and each part evolves to a higher level.

In posture work, learn how to be still, to see which parts need to be stretched and which parts need to emphasize straightness. If the legs are wobbly or spine wrongly shaped, concentrating on keeping them firm and straight whenever possible throughout the day will eventually establish a new character in them. Parts such as the pelvic area and shoulders may need to be given careful attention, relaxation and exercise before they will truly respond and be receptive to your love. Observe any reactions without identifying with them.

In life look at the position of your affairs by asking, "What is the situation?" "What needs to be done and how can I do it in a way that fits the situation and at the same time gives fulfillment?" SEE WHAT IS REAL, WHAT IS NOT REAL, WHAT IS IN ACCORD WITH THE TRUE BEING.

PART 4

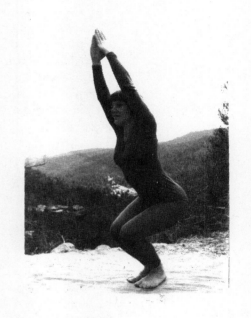

BODY-MIND AS ONE WHOLE

PRACTICAL SITUATION – SELF CONFRONTATION

Either: a) Fast for one whole day,

b) Keep silence as much as possible both externally and internally for one day,

c) Be completely alone for one or two days eating only a light diet and doing no-thing.

Choose whichever of the above situations is practical for you and do it as sensibly as possible, without imposing it upon others or making it difficult for those you live with. Ask them when it will be convenient for you to "have a day off" for this work on yourself. Find a time and a place so that you can apply yourself whole-heartedly to this session with yourself!

During the session:

1) Look back over your life and look at what character-istics you see to be of your higher self. Perhaps the abili-ty to organize or to be creative; perhaps a love of people or the love of life itself. Perhaps there were certain times when you took responsibility and now you see that it was right to do so.

2) Look next at what you see to be your lower self. Perhaps certain bad habits; perhaps certain thoughts. Perhaps you feel that at sometime past you have been wrongly judged and you have let your mind become bitter or resentful. Or perhaps you are allowing too much resistance to certain changes you need to make.

3) Look at the one who is seeing these opposite sides of yourself. Go back in your life to your earliest recollec-tions and see if you can identify with a state of consciousness that is unchanged by your life experiences.

4) Look at those actions and states of consciousness that brought about a good effect ultimately, even though at that time it may have been painful. Ask about each action and the consciousness associated with it:

IS THIS ME?

IS THIS NOT ME?

WHAT IS THE TRUE REALITY?

Ask also "Do I really want to change? Why?" Be honest with yourself at all times, otherwise life may later reflect back dishonesty when it is not so easy to accept as now.

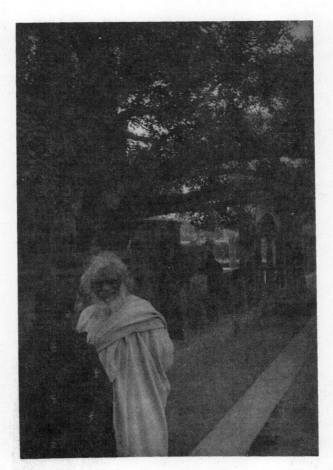

Photograph taken by Christopher Hills at the Bo Tree where Buddha was enlightened 2,500 years ago. The Holy Man traveled with Christopher Hills all over India.

STUDY MATERIAL
SUMMARY OF SECTION 1

So far we have been studying consciousness by questioning ourself and whatever we see consciously around us. The answers to such questions as "What is consciousness, and why study it?" were expanded and it is for each individual to test and apply these answers in his or her own life. To summarize:

Consciousness is what we see with and what is seen. Consciousness is life energy, vibrating with awareness and moved by a motivating will power (Life Force).

The nature of consciousness is to express itself through polarity and diversity and to experience itself through unity and relativity.

The function of consciousness is to balance its inherent forces and evolve natural patterns of life energy that are a reflection of itself.

Laws of consciousness state that:

> Consciousness goes where it is directed.
>
> Consciousness sees only what is of itself.
>
> Consciousness evolves according to the interest in it and by the willingness to grow from it.

The way in which we recognize the source of the self -- SELF-REALIZATION -- is by learning the ways (laws) of consciousness, and applying them. Both in growth practices -- such as yoga, meditation, encounter work, etc. -- and in the actual practical situations of life, Self-realization can be attained. Without this realization, life can be uncertain and confusing. With this realization, direction and certainty can bring all things to their natural fruition.

To do anything there must be love. A love of truth and understanding is the highest form of love. Throughout the ages great masters have sought to communicate this love to those who have been ready to receive the ultimate gift of knowing themselves. In appreciation, the chosen ones have taken on a discipleship, a bond of love, which has freed them from the bonds of delusion and liberated them into a state of enlightenment, a state of seeing things clearly; as they really are.

A disciple becomes a master by practising a discipline -- an act of love -- until there is no separation between the Self-contact of the master and the Self-contact of the disciple. A disciple of Life becomes at one with life itself when he can discipline all energies within him to the extent that life creates no barriers for him and he creates no resistance to the flow of energy through him. He and the universe are then as ONE. He is then in tune with God.

Self-discipline is the finest discipline and the only discipline ultimately. Though one may surrender to the guidance of someone who has "trodden the path", in order to save incarnations of going up blind alleys, Self effort and study are still the requirements of any earnest student. Sometimes the influence of someone with a stronger bond of fellowship with Truth can induce a large flow of energy if and when the student is ready to receive it. However, direct initiation is by God for all who seek with the willingness and patience to discipline their consciousness towards a greater self-awareness and self-development.

In this course one is learning how to be guided by life and to discipline consciousness accordingly, rather than seeing Truth only, for example, through body discipline or religious devotion. Though each section of this course emphasizes a particular area of consciousness (body, mind or soul), these areas are looked at as a mirror of the whole. Hence evolution in the mentality may reflect an increase in the quality of expression through the body and expansion of love from the soul, shown as an ability to relate to more of life at a deeper level of understanding. Similarly, evolution of the physical level may reflect an increase in mental stamina and a radiance of the soul that can be seen in the eyes.

A basic discipline for self-knowledge through life is to:

> Observe all things without judging. Listen
> to what life is saying without assuming
> what should or ought to be done.

> Inquire within,
> "What is the real situation?"
> "What do I see as most important and
> what has to be done?"
> "How can I best fulfill the need of the
> moment?"

> Learn how to experience and move conscious-
> ness willingly, cheerfully, with direction
> and with certainty.

Any kind of true discipline is one in which there is a willing response to the master. Life is a master and if we bear any resentments or grievances about how life is treating us, it is no different from bearing them against a personal master. A true master's discipline can be just as severe as some of life's lessons. If we are to accept the love that a master or life gives, we must also accept the hardships. However, these are not really hardships when we see the beauty of a refined consciousness with control, sensitivity, and deep love, devoid of aggression or rigidity. There is a guideline in the saying "Use your common sense." What is meant of course is to see things from a pure sense, with intelligence and an understanding of what is natural. What is natural is a balance and a moderation in all things.

Discipline therefore becomes a balancing and a purifying of energies: putting things in their rightful place and letting go of any reactions of the body or any thoughts and feelings of the mind. If one day is spent eating too much or worrying about food, then balance it with a day of fasting, with the consciousness more on the spirit of life. If the mind has been roaming aimlessly, spend time focussing the consciousness on something worthwhile.

Conscious direction with a feeling for living and a more aware state of consciousness is discipline. Austerities are not always necessary but awareness and a conscious balancing are very important. The difference between a master and a student is that a master sees when he needs to eat and he eats. When he sits in meditation he meditates. A student thinks about eating when he meditates and tries to meditate when he is eating. Nevertheless, it is necessary to become a student before one can become a master. To realize this is to become humble and to become humble is to become pure.*

See with a pure heart and love is a natural outpouring. Discipline can then be applied without thought of it as a discipline but as an act of love. In training oneself to become an ever more open channel of life energy, one is growing in love power. In learning to attune to the real need of the moment one is growing in awareness and one will soon see with the wisdom of a master and acquire an everlasting bond of love with the master of life itself.

* The taped lecture on "Self-Mastery" from the "Speak to us of . . . " series by Christopher Hills is a recommended supplement to this section. This two-cassette lecture is available from the University of the Trees Press. See the tape list at the rear of this book for details.

DAILY PRACTICE FOR PART 4

THEME:
DIRECTION COMES THROUGH RIGHT LEARNING
DISCIPLINE FOLLOWS FROM A CARING EFFORT

Let yesterday's truth be only a memory for the recurring patterns of life to be observed. Live for today and be open to new learning. Through a giving to life and a seeking only after greater self-knowledge, a deeper understanding will come.

In facing today's truth and mastering its message, life will reveal the reason for the past and a direction for the future, which will ultimately unfold if the direction is followed. One may then receive the state of grace which the Tao describes as a state of "doing without doing". In this state of consciousness which is pure, rewards are not necessary for work done. Work is indeed joy in itself. Perhaps you have sometimes experienced this joy with work that is fulfilling for you. Perhaps you know of the real contentment that comes from such action.

POSTURE PRACTICE

Notice the effects of postures. Feel and see how:

STANDING POSTURES uplift the consciousness and give stability.

BALANCING POSTURES make the consciousness receptive and sensitive to movement.

INVERTED POSTURES introvert the consciousness and promote spiritual strength.

BACKBENDING POSTURES make the consciousness more active and encourage vitality.

TWISTING POSTURES broaden the consciousness and stimulate a changing field of activity.

FORWARD-BENDING POSTURES make the consciousness more passive and calm the nerves and emotions.

UPWARD-SITTING POSTURES build a strong mind and an attuned state of consciousness.

LYING POSTURES still the consciousness and promote awareness of the silent center within.

Diagram 4.1.

ARROWS ⟶ depict effect of postures on the direction of consciousness

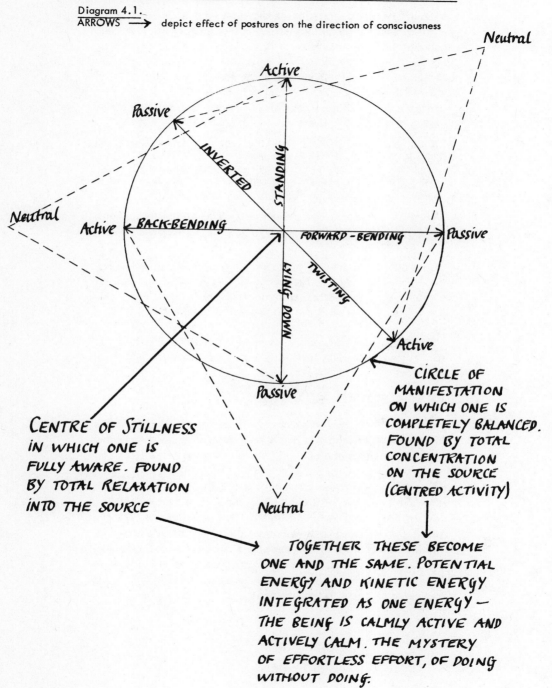

CENTRE OF STILLNESS IN WHICH ONE IS FULLY AWARE. FOUND BY TOTAL RELAXATION INTO THE SOURCE

CIRCLE OF MANIFESTATION ON WHICH ONE IS COMPLETELY BALANCED. FOUND BY TOTAL CONCENTRATION ON THE SOURCE (CENTRED ACTIVITY)

TOGETHER THESE BECOME ONE AND THE SAME. POTENTIAL ENERGY AND KINETIC ENERGY INTEGRATED AS ONE ENERGY — THE BEING IS CALMLY ACTIVE AND ACTIVELY CALM. THE MYSTERY OF EFFORTLESS EFFORT, OF DOING WITHOUT DOING.

Determine the center line of the body and work towards an even balance of consciousness at either side of it. Keep the consciousness at either side of it. Keep the consciousness lifting up the front of the body and down the back. Broaden equally across the front of the body and at the back of the body.

In each posture find a position of balance in which you are at ease.

Keep the body still but aim the consciousness towards the perfect posture.

When the body becomes restless move the negative restless energy with a positive direction into the perfect posture.

Then be still again. Breathe smoothly and evenly throughout.

Observe on the inhalation and stretch on the exhalation.

Continue this practice until there is a continuous steady movement towards the perfect posture with the consciousness completely at ease. When there is strain, be still, or move to a counter posture or relax out of the posture completely.

Remember the body is like a person. Relate to it as such. Be firm but not aggressive, be flexible but not a slave to it.

PRANAYAM: HEALTH THROUGH BREATH

Breathing is one way in which we vibrate our consciousness. The most natural breathing is like a sine wave; even, with an equal inhalation to exhalation.

Discriminate between drawing the breath into the lungs and allowing it to flow in. Combine the two so that there is neither a forcing nor a lagging in the breath. This is the attuned state in which the individual is breathing at the same rate as the natural rhythm, programed by the universe at that time. The individual and the universe are then as one and there is no discrimination between I and IT. No-thing and every-thing are the same thing and peace describes this attunement.

Diagram 4.2.

COMBINATION OF AWARENESS
AND ENERGY IN TUNED
STATE OF BALANCE

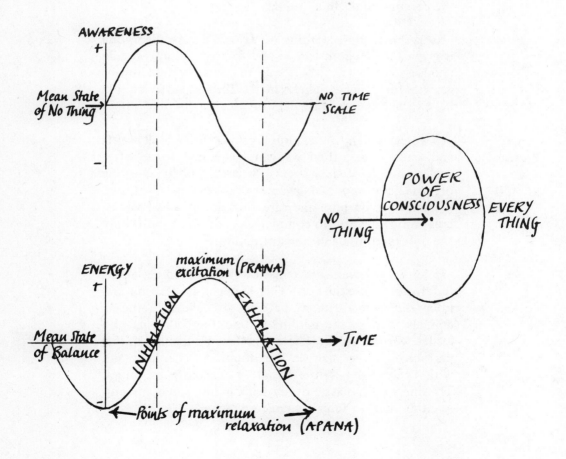

AWARENESS

Mean State of No Thing → NO TIME SCALE

POWER OF CONSCIOUSNESS

NO THING → · EVERY THING

ENERGY

maximum excitation (PRANA)

Mean State of Balance → TIME

INHALATION   EXHALATION

Points of maximum relaxation (APANA)

93

APPLICATION TO LIFE

The whole of creation, plantlife, animal nature, human behavior and other aspects of consciousness, can all be understood by examining the movements of our own individual consciousness which has evolved through the various stages of growth to the present human form. The next stage of growth is to be aware of the many aspects of creation within our own consciousness, then to expand with this light of awareness, and experience the common links in all things.

Everything acts according to its own nature. Everyone is given the freedom to live and to grow in any way he chooses. However, if that way restricts the freedom of growth for others, then events, pain and suffering will be experienced as a signal for change to take place.

If we can listen to what life is saying through all events and experiences, then we can be guided to a better understanding of the effects of our actions, the meaning of true love and add awareness of the giver of life. Guided by a purpose and direction in life, each part of creation can evolve to complement and assist more fully the process of life and transformation.

In all living organisms, consciousness is feeding, and is fed from, consciousness. This happens in relating and integrating the different patterns of behavior. Among animals there is the herding instinct,the following of a leader who brings the whole together. With some animal partnerships the male is the dominant character and with other animals, the female is in charge of things. The one who is master of himself can have predominantly either male or female characteristics.

With plants too there are those that harmonize and those, like certain weeds, that choke the growth of the other plants around them. Some people choke other people's lives, and need to live in an environment where they can grow in their own way and learn self-control without imposing upon the freedom of others. Nevertheless, what one man calls a weed may be a useful herb, or a beautiful flower to another. The viewpoint may change, but the situation and results of the nature of things may not be so easy to change. In groups of people some can be treated with kindness and they will respond to it. Some need a "kick up the backside" before they will respond to what needs to be done.

Life displays many patterns according to the situation. By integrating and not interfering, we can assist the whole process of evolution. Learn the nature of things and see the situation as it really is. This gives the direction. Assist according to the real need, and a love of the source is made manifest. Evolution is then certain and peace is the reward.

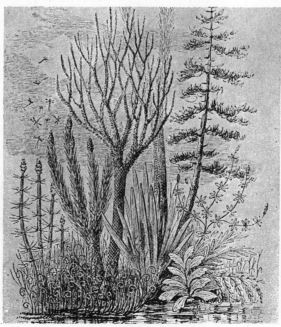

SECTION 2

This section develops the practices of Section 1 further to a deeper level. The consciousness is directed into looking at what is behind the physical world. That is, a looking at the mind and the invisible forces that determine the physical manifestation, also turning mental states into physical realities and physical actions into psychological patterns that harmonize with the true nature of man. More time is given to precision in postures, to sensing the details of experience and to increasing the awareness of the subtleties of relationships.

In brief: Levels of consciousness,

              Mind energy flow,

              Seeing the mind with the body.

* Much of Sections 2 and 3 is based on the work of Christopher Hills, gleaned from oral, written and taped teachings. The seven levels of consciousness and their relationship to color and light is taken from original research by Christopher Hills, written about extensively in his book "Nuclear Evolution: Discovery of the Rainbow Body."

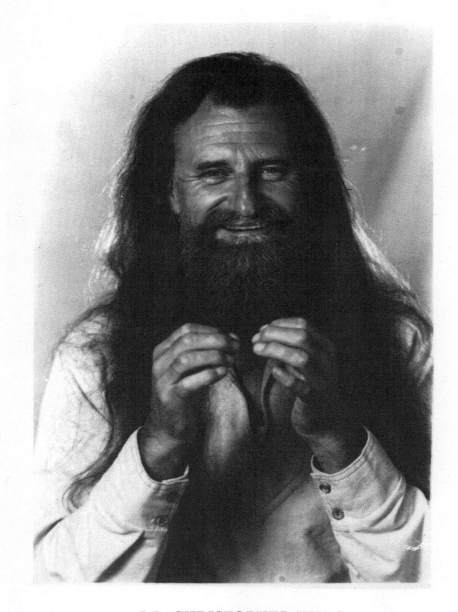

DR. CHRISTOPHER HILLS
Author of "Nuclear Evolution:
Discovery of the Rainbow Body"

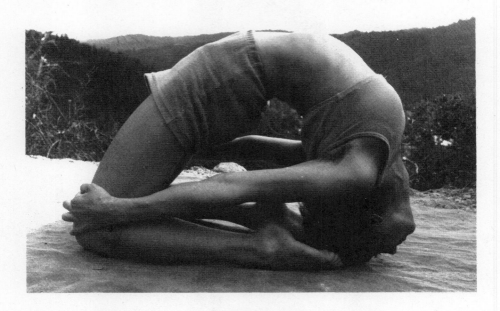

LAGHURAJRASANA

To live is to learn and to go where one is.
To love is to give and to receive what one has.
Loving and learning of what is given already,
How often do we look to the one who is steady?
Look to the ONE and all things will be revealed,
Be centered in the ONE and all longings will be sealed.

PART 5

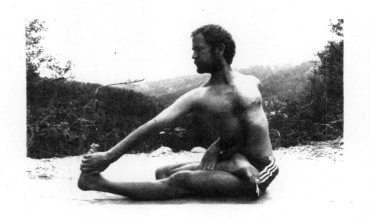

SEVEN THRESHOLDS OF NUCLEAR EVOLUTION AND THE WHOLE BEING

PRACTICAL SITUATION --- SELF ANALYSIS

Set aside one whole day in which to concentrate on this exercise.

PROCEDURE

Record, either verbally onto a tape recorder, or in writing, the thoughts that are passing through your mind during the day. Do this from say 9 a.m. to 5 p.m., recording or writing the thoughts on each hour and half-hour of the clock. Be as lucid as possible and as honest as possible.

If you have a very trusting friend who is also doing this course you could do this individually and then together discuss the effects of it upon each of you. However, make sure that inside of you both, there is a bond of love that accepts each other unconditionally, whatever tendencies you may need to work through in the consciousness. Remember that true love lies beyond all positive and negative actions and reactions.

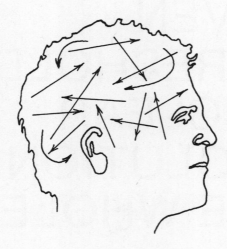

ANALYSIS

Analyze your thoughts alone as they were recorded. They may range from, perhaps, philosophical arguments with yourself, to domestic matters or even sexual fantasies. Be as objective as possible in your observations and examine what came into the consciousness and how it came in. What caused it? Are there any recurring thought patterns? Do they spring from a conditioning in childhood? In your work during this day did your thoughts relate to whatever you were doing or did they spin around in a world of their own? Compare how you experienced it at that time and now in retrospect.

See if you can see the cause of your thinking. What are true wholesome patterns of thought and what are draining you of energy or taking you away from your true center? Understand what is your true center and put your thoughts on THAT.

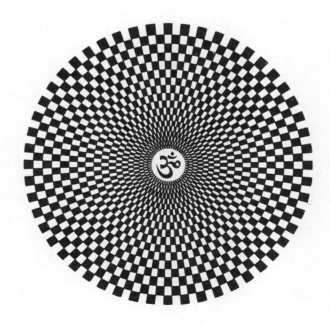

STUDY MATERIAL

LEVELS OF CONSCIOUSNESS

The laws of consciousness, the nature of consciousness and the functions of it that apply to everyday experience were examined in Section 1. Diagram 5.1 shows seven psychological layers of consciousness and drives associated with the seven main body functions. In Section 2 we are going to look at these areas of consciousness and in particular the reasoning faculty of the intellect, the feeling quality of the mind, the conceptualizing or associating part of our thought processes and the intuitive faculty of direct knowing through the psyche.

The "mind-stuff" is a field of vibrating energy patterns. Even the body is a function of the mind: it is condensed mind-stuff. The effect of intense concentration and identification of the ego with form over a period of millions of years has established man's thought patterns in a physical reality that is dependent upon the thought process and is therefore not SELF existent. The true Being is beyond or behind not only the physical state but also the mind state. However it is through these planes of consciousness that we are able to experience different dimensions of consciousness and see their nature as a description of pure consciousness. In each level, the reality of pure consciousness, of eternal SELF existence, is maintaining the stream of conscious vibration from which each plane is developed. Like the carrier wave of a television waveform that contains many frequencies within it, pure consciousness has inherent within it all states of consciousness.

We can tune into this all-pervading stream of vibration through meditation and hear the wide range of sounds (called the OM sound) on physical to psychic levels.

Now just as we can tune to a wide band of frequencies with a television receiver and yet tune to a specific program frequency, so it is with consciousness. When we tune our television set to a frequency of, for example, 96 megacycles, we receive signals of sound, picture, synchronizing pulses and many more waveforms, each of which contains its own particular piece of information that goes to make up the whole presentation of the TV program.

It is the structure of the TV set and the alignment of the circuitry that enables the analysis and synthesis of the program material to be presented on the screen.

In the structuring of consciousness, the body, mind and soul are used to analyze and synthesize the stream of pure consciousness to show the program of life through the functions of various body centers, mind patterns and psychological drives. The cause and manifestation of these vibrations or levels of consciousness are the study of meditation and of this course.

The seven physical functions of consciousness explained in Section 1 could be looked at as energy manifested on different levels in a vertical sense. The seven psychological drives depicted in diagram 5.1. below could be looked at as energy manifested on different levels in a horizontal sense. Since the body is a manifestation of the finer vibrations of the mind, each level of the mind has a corresponding area of the body which displays the nature and characteristics of that level.

The diagram following shows these areas and the associated level of consciousness from the psychological viewpoint.

Diagram 5.1.

HILLS' LEVELS OF CONSCIOUSNESS

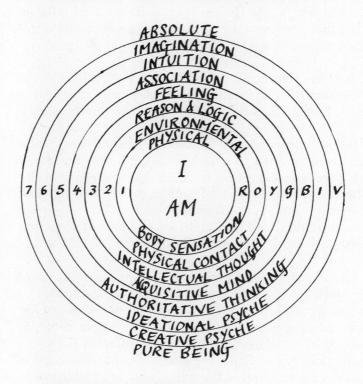

RESONANT COLOR

R – Red
O – Orange
Y – Yellow
G – Green

B – Blue
I – Indigo
V – Violet

Area of Body	Part of Spinal Column	Gland	Psychological Drive
Head	Cerebrum	Pineal	Imaginative
Face	Cerebellum	Pituitary	Intuitive
Neck	Cervical	Thyroid	Conceptual
Chest & Arms	Dorsal	Thymus	Security
Middle	Lumbar	Pancreas	Intellectual
Waist	Sacral	Adrenal	Social
Legs	Coccyx	Gonads	Physical

Each psychological drive has associated with it certain characteristics in the consciousness, such as the way time is experienced and the way that the positive and negative aspects of consciousness are expressed. A person who functions mostly on the intellectual level likes to reason everything out and put things in definite categories. He experiences each event with a past, present and future, according to a set of conditions. If this reasoning proves to be in accord with true facts, then he experiences a sense of attunement with his reasoning faculty.

If someone comes up with a fact, let us say, from the intuition, which he knows without knowing why he knows it, then his logic is challenged and he may feel uncomfortable to the extent that he becomes argumentative and possibly irate or even aggressive.

This is the problem of seeing only from one level. It is the cause of poor communication and many unhappy relationships. If we can learn to see on other levels and experience from other viewpoints, we are at a definite advantage for knowing the whole SELF and relating with others. The seven main psychological drives and the basic need of each level are shown in the table that follows.

Since each level of consciousness is a vibration, each resonates with related frequencies in other octaves of the total frequency spectrum. In his book *Nuclear Evolution: Discovery of the Rainbow Body* Christopher Hills shows how each level of consciousness resonates with one of the seven main colors of the rainbow and one of the seven fundamental sound frequencies. He also shows how color affects the consciousness and stimulates the various drives and needs. A summary of these findings is given in the table on the following pages.

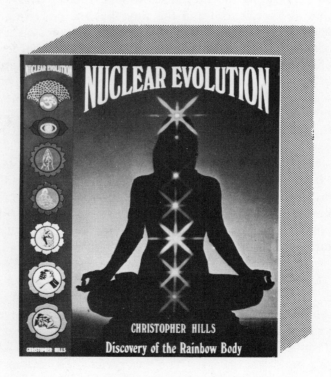

Color	Drive	Experience of Time	Consciousness
Red	Self-replication	Present	*Need for activity* and body sensation. Likes to get things done now. However, not always aware of the importance of careful thinking and the effect of his actions on the future.
Orange	Herd Instinct	Future & Present	*Need for social contact.* Ambitious, likes to share sense pleasure with others. Makes others feel physically satisfied but sometimes forgets that there is work to be done on other levels.
Yellow	Intellect	Past, Present & Future	*Need for change.* Sees situations as mathematical problems with answers worked out by reason. Categorizes and is good at planning but is not easily sensitive to other's feelings.
Green	Acquisitive	Past, Present or Future	*Need for security.* Describes life through feelings. Has a sense of responsibility and is usually good at handling money. However, easily jealous of others. Is wary of "taking the plunge".
Blue	Conceptual	Past	*Need for authority.* Sensitive, Idealist and family orientated. Likes harmony at all costs. Therefore sometimes rejects anything unconventional or uncomfortable.
Indigo	Intuition	Future	*Need for contemplation.* Works everything out through ideas in the mind, seeing it all complete in the future, but finds difficulty in manifesting the ideas on the physical level in the present.
Violet	Imagination	Past, Present & Future	*Need for freedom.* Thinks, fancies and senses with new concepts and creativity. Likes order out of chaos. However, does not easily accept criticism and finds it hard to face the reality here and now. This world is one of mystery, magic and charm.

LIVING YOGA

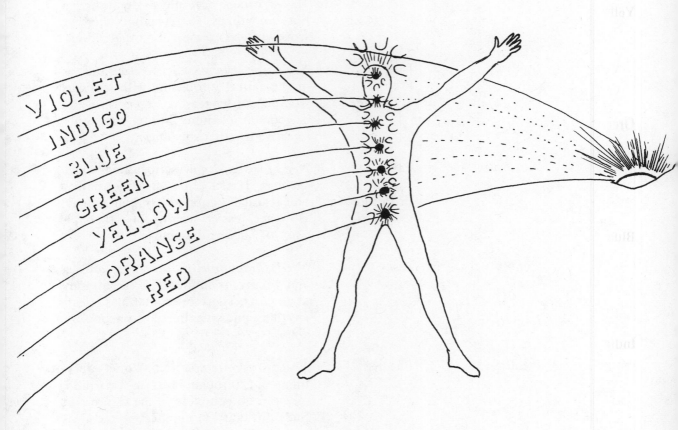

VIOLET
INDIGO
BLUE
GREEN
YELLOW
ORANGE
RED

The table of psychological drives could be represented as a double pyramid as shown in the diagram 5.2. This diagram is merely a representation to show that in each state of consciousness there are ascending and descending levels. Levels below one's normal level of operations can usually be more easily understood than those above. A person who is enveloped in the physical world will not easily see the poetical expanded consciousness of the person who is on the imagination level, whereas the person with imagination can more readily put himself into the "inner world" or mind of a physical person and at least have some idea of his experience. However, the absolute is in all things and as shown in the diagram, to be centered

Diagram 5.2.

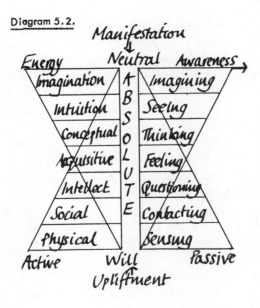

in any one level brings an understanding of the problems of life and the realization of Truth on any other level. You will see that the active, passive and neutral elements, the universal triune of forces (three gunas) is also working on all levels so that it is not necessarily easier to reach the absolute from one level than from another. Total fulfillment comes when there can be understanding from the viewpoint of each level. Remember here that "level" refers to a vibratory rate and not to any superior quality or ability. Each level has its function in the same way as the organs and glands of the body have theirs. Just as a developed brain without a body through which to experess its development is of little use, so the imagination without feelings and thoughts through which to express the images is of little value.

You will notice from the previous table of the levels of consciousness that there are certain levels seemingly with the same time world. In fact this is not so. The past, present and future of the yellow intellect is experienced in linear form with a sequential ordering of events. The past, present and future of the green heart level is one in which an experience of, for instance, owning something is enjoyed in the now from the point of view of security (car, money, loved one). When the object of possession is experienced, dreams of its future use or development give one an interest in the future, because of what one has now. If the object is lost or taken away, then the memory of what one had in the past is important and fills the consciousness.

The past, present and future of the violet imagination is eternal time in which everything is seen in "spaced out" cosmic terms. Life is a drama or a fantasy and what is now is present everywhere. The sound of leaves rustling together is the sound of life moving with the tide of time. Wars of the past are echoed in the thunder of a storm and a future world of perfection is only a

110

few lifetimes away. This is the world of someone who lives mainly in the imaginative state of consciousness. Compare this with the very practical red level person who wants to do things now and to see it happening now. Can you see what might happen when one person on the imaginative level and one on the physical level are together in a room? If someone knocks on the door the imaginative person may describe the sound by saying, "Hark, I hear the Cosmic Heartbeat," and will wait for an echo of it. To the physical level person that is ridiculous; there is someone knocking at the door and he goes to let him in. The violet level person knows there is someone at the door but heard the knock possibly in terms of how he might hear the knock from the eternal one who brings enlightenment. The physical person simply sees things with the senses and does not choose to experience the dreamlike state which the violet level person enjoys. However, he does enjoy being practical and down to earth, which the violet level person finds very difficult. Hence the latter may become confused or overburdened when the car breaks down or the house needs a spring cleaning. Chaos breaks out and outside help from a mechanic or domestic help is often the only answer.

The future of the orange social drive is again quite different from that of the indigo level. The orange level person is an organizer, but in the not-too-distant future, and he is concerned mainly with physical or sense well-being. He sees the future from the point of view of present and past experience.

The future of the indigo intuitive drive is based on the faculty of intuiting (knowing without knowing why one knows) as he is not too concerned about past or present but mainly with ideas and happenings that bring absolute perfection into his life. He sees patterns of the future in terms of a person's inner state or depth of knowing rather than the orange person's manifested welfare state for humanity's social needs.

Emotions come from a level between green and blue, like the color of sea water. Emotions fluctuate between the melancholy and upliftment of the blue level and the excitement and love of life on the green level.

The past of the blue conceptual person is a memory of associations, and present events are compared with the events of history. Hence this person and the futuristic person of the indigo level are seeing the present situation in quite different ways. It can be very difficult for both of them to see the NOW without any reference to time. Therefore to learn to see it AS IT IS NOW with the possibility that IT MAY STAY THIS WAY FOREVER OR CHANGE IN THE NEXT INSTANT would be a good exercise for people in both blue and indigo areas.

Relationships are useful in understanding these levels and hence the nature of consciousness. This means that one needs to practice becoming the person that one is relating to. To do this, one needs to appreciate the inner world of another, recognizing in oneself the way that energy is moving and to go with the positive flow that centers the consciousness of the other person in oneself. If the person is dreaming, help him or her to dream of how to tackle the practical problems of the moment and to see them through. This needs skill; interfering or "trying to help" can cause resentment in the other person rather than gratitude. It is better first to experience a person and to observe the effects of the experience. Then, with discrimination, one acknowledges what appears to be in order and sees how what appears to be at fault came into consciousness.

The body is a map of consciousness and all the levels can be seen manifested in the body. Tension in the shoulders has its origin in the emotions. Ulcers in the stomach have their causation in the social and intellectual responsibilities. The action of the arms is the manifestation of the heart's love of giving and of acquiring for one's security the feeling of belonging. (The throat allows the voicing of authority on the blue level.) When this authority is challenged, it can bring a lump in the throat. When there is a centeredness the throat can be the channel for a clear expression of the Truth. The future of the indigo person manifests as a **higher** forehead as he looks ahead to the future. Problems in the legs and hips are problems on the red and orange level. A body with no problems shows a clear mind and a balance of the various energies on all levels. A person in this highly developed state can offer that perfection to others and in the process can gain further understanding, since consciousness is ever feeding off consciousness and evolving as a whole to a new order of Self awareness and Self expression.

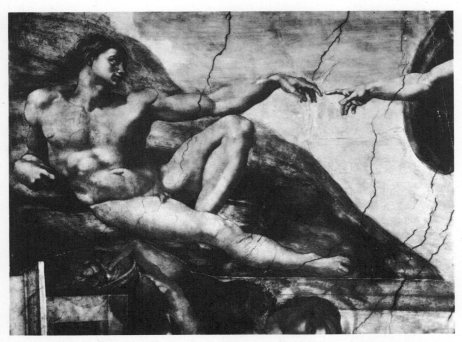

Michaelangelo's concept of a perfect body is shown in this detail of the picture on p. 64 of the body of Adam being created by the power of God, or Consciousness. Man's fall from this perfection is symbolized by his banishment from the effortless garden of Eden, where God and man were an extension and expression of each other.

113

DAILY PRACTICE FOR PART 5

THEME:
LOOK NOT FOR THAT WHICH CAN BE SEEN WITH
THE EYES
BUT SEARCH FOR THE ONE WHO IS CONSCIOUS
WITH NO "I".

In all practices, observation, self-analysis an awareness of the true self is essential. Senses, thoughts and feelings can easily seek stimulation and cause man to become identified with the impermanent world of sensations, intellectual planning and comfortable idealism. Sensations, thinking processes and loves of the heart are very powerful forces and cannot be ignored. To reject them is to suppress an urge for expression. However, it is not wise to let them dominate or be completely loose when concern and effort can channel that energy into a wholesome fulfillment from within.

The first thing to realize is that the same one who is looking outwards can also look inwards to "THE ONE who is looking" in all directions. All selves come from the one Self and therefore an urge to express love can be channelled towards a person, into an idea or into an action. It can also be channelled into pure devotion to the Source which created the means for expression in the first place. When one is completely absorbed in a state of love or in the essence of an action, then joy comes. For instance, if you go fishing to catch fish but catch none, you are disappointed. But if you go with no expectations, you enjoy the fishing whether you catch anything or not.

POSTURE PRACTICE:
POSE AND COUNTERPOSE

One way of understanding pose and counterpose is to relate positions of the body to situations in life. What position (state of consciousness) are we in now? What positions do we put ourselves into? Look at the sequence of decisions that bring repeated cycles of events into your life. The ability to move consciousness and to change position, literally outwardly or inwardly, needs the skill of the same "I" that is as conscious of day-to-day activity as it is when doing yoga postures.

114

The body too is a reflection of our Consciousness expressing all levels of our nature. The legs and pelvic area show the physical qualities and the nature of their expression; the trunk outlines the mental capacities and the head displays the soul attributes and qualities. When you look into someone's eyes deeply do you see their soul nature? Watch the way you hold your own body when you tackle a problem and you will see the dynamics of your own mind. See how people who stand really firmly on their legs have physical stamina in their day to day work. Body, mind and soul are only degrees of the one conscious life energy that flows through all things. Nature is constantly balancing its movements of energy. The cycles of day and night, spring, summer, autumn and winter give an indication of a natural process of attunement between the parts of creation and a still center of total awareness and infinite potential energy. If one has lost contact with this center of creation, the re-searching and experimenting are necessary requirements of life. Hence Yoga!

For a study of the effects of body positioning and conscious movement see how in standing upright, the upliftment of the body and therefore of consciousness encourages confidence and stability. Likewise, in tackling a physical job in life, can you take the same approach? How do you feel when you have done a lot of physical work? Tired? Depressed? Isn't the natural desire to put your feet up and find inner contentment, and rejuvenate by relaxing? In Hatha Yoga we do this too: every pose has its counterpose; every state of mind has its counteracting state. After putting consciousness into the soul with the headstand and feeding it with spiritual energy, then naturally we look to a means of expressing it. Notice the expressiveness of a backbend such as chakrasana. Experiment further, then ask:

a) What are the positive effects in the consciousness of each of the seven main types of postures (standing, inverted, backbends, twists, forward bends, lying on the back and sitting)?

b) Doing the postures in the order above, do you sense a feeling of balance? of pose and counterpose?

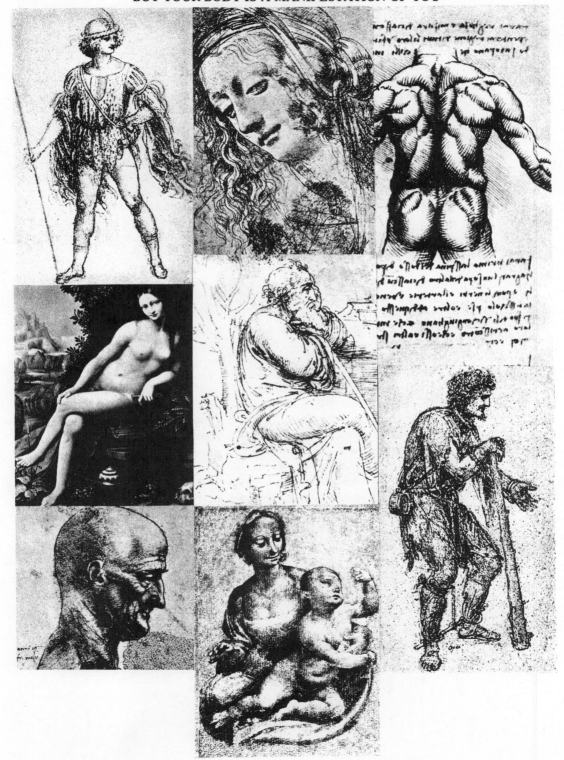

PRANAYAM --- HEALTH THROUGH BREATH
ENERGIZING BREATH
Using Khumbaka (breath retention)

1) Sit upright, either in Virasana, Padmasana or some other comfortable sitting posture. Sitting on a chair is acceptable as long as you can sit for some time with the sacrum lifting the spine upright and straight and the collarbone horizontal to the ground with the shoulders well back.

2) Breathe as you did in Section 1 through the nostrils and the throat, into the lungs and out again in a smooth, even manner.

3) Become aware of the expansion of the lungs internally, with very little movement of the body. Keep the shoulders still and hold the rib cage in a fully opened condition with the floating ribs well separated from the pelvic rim.

4) Exhale completely and wait for the breath to come in.

5) Inhale in attunement with the breath as learned in Section 1, taking eight beats to full inhalation. Make sure that both lungs are filling evenly and feel a broadening of the body as the breath enters the lungs.

6) Hold for eight beats keeping the height of the chest and keeping the consciousness centered in the fullness of the breath.

7) Exhale for eight beats, lifting the front of the arm pits and feeling a dropping of the skin and shoulderblades down the back. Draw in the stomach slightly at the end of the exhalation and wait in the stillness for the next breath to come in. Listen to the silence with the consciousness centered on contentment.

8) Repeat the breathing cycle increasing the ratio to 10:10:10 after you are able to repeat 8:8:8 ratio for at least five minutes. Never increase the ratio unless you can maintain it for at least five minutes without any sign of lung strain. Do not hold the breath if you have high blood pressure.

N.B. After all breathing exercises, relax and meditate by becoming very still and listening to any sound that comes into the consciousness. Let go of anything that tries to disturb the serenity and stillness of the state of pure consciousness. If you cannot let go of disturbances, look for the cause of the disturbances. Relax and meditate.

See how you can use the results of your research on Pose and Counterpose in life. For example, what is the Counterpose for too much bending over a typewriter or sink?

See if you can notice in what area people are functioning and discover how to communicate with them on their level. For example, a person who says "I think" is on a thinking level, a person who says "I feel" is on a feeling level. See how you can put yourself into their "world" and think or feel with them.

APPLICATION TO LIFE

See how you can use the results of your research on Pose and Counterpose in life. For example, what is the Counterpose for too much bending over a typewriter or sink?

See if you can notice in what area people are functioning and discover how to communicate with them on their level. For example, a person who says "I think" is on a thinking level; a person who says "I feel" is on a feeling level. See how you can put yourself into their "world" and think or feel with them.

PART 6

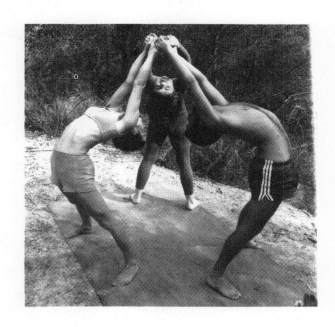

A HEALTHY BALANCE OF THE FUNDAMENTAL ENERGIES OF THE WHOLE MAN

PRACTICAL SITUATION --- SELF LOVE

As with all these practical situations we are dealing with life as it confronts us and we experience it in our consciousness. Consciousness is conditioned by what is put into it and the amount of attachment to this conditioning is the feedback of this session.

In the state of pure consciousness there is no attachment, since there is nothing to be attached to except existence and on all levels the giving of consciousness is a giving of the SELF to the SELF through some form of love. In pure love there is no separation between giver and receiver. Love gives and love receives as an expression of its SELF. Pure love is a very high state of consciousness to experience and yet it can be achieved.

EXERCISE

a) Expand your consciousness to feel yourself in all things. Start with the consciousness in the heart and concentrate on the beat of the heart. Feel the heartbeat throughout the body from the toes to the top of the head. Feel yourself in another person and see if you can sense their heartbeat. Feel yourself in plants, the walls of the room, the environment, and in the sky and the fields.

If you can find someone to do the exercise with you, face each other, and look into the eyes. Send love out from the heart. Feel the heart energy of the other person without desire or attachment to it. Simply receive and enjoy it as a gift of cosmic love from the life-giver who is inside of you. Similarly, allow the same life force to flow freely from your heart to the other person and see it coming back to you out of the eyes of the other person as another part of yourself. If you wish, discuss the experience and say what you saw in the eyes of the other person. Did you see your higher SELF?

b) Ask yourself honestly and sincerely:

    1) "What is security for me?"
    2) "What possession do I value most?"
    Meditate on or discuss these questions with your friend openly.

c) Test your green level strength by seeing if you can let go of one of your prized possessions and securities. For example, can you do without your car, a certain comforting habit, financial reward or emotional support when work is done? Can you be without the presence of a loving partner? Or harder still, can you let go of your thoughts?

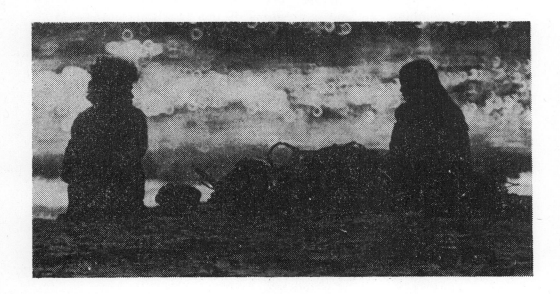

STUDY MATERIAL

EXPRESSION AND RECEPTIVITY

In all levels of consciousness there is a central state of pure consciousness that cannot be described or defined. Each level of consciousness is a field of energy, vibrating consciously at a certain rate. It arises out of, and ultimately returns to, its pure state. Waves rise from a still lake on a stormy day and return to a state of peace and tranquility when the disturbance has subsided. This is the nature of consciousness.

Different rates and combinations of vibrations give rise to different characteristics in the waveform of consciousness and these manifest as diversity, polarity and individuality. To understand consciousness fully, experience of the pure state and of the characteristics of the different levels is necessary since life consists of combinations and expressions of the basic characteristics of all the levels.

All states and levels of consciousness come originally from a still state and find fulfillment in a balancing of polarity (positive/negative, male/female, active/passive) so that expression and a reflection of that expression are seen and experienced in ever new ways.

The relationships with one's own body, mind and soul, and with others, all help us to gain an understanding of the levels of consciousness, the nature of their characteristics, and the feeling of the presence of the ONE SELF that originally created them.

Energy goes where the heart is, while the head provides an objective channel of awareness to view its movements. The reasoning power of the intellect is often considered a male attribute and the feeling of the heart a female tendency. In fact, all levels of consciousness are encompassed in male and female alike and the true heart, the spiritual heart, is neither male nor female.

This heart of the being draws energy from the physical, mental and psychic reservoirs of the all-pervading cosmic energy. The universal forces of attraction and repulsion direct the cosmic energy through a set of invisible frequency-discriminating centers called Chakras, into the psychic, mental and physical realms of Individualized consciousness.

Chakras are wheels of energy generated by fundamental frequencies in the universal spectrum of vibration. These fundamental vibrations create in the consciousness energy patterns such as the natural smooth wave-like form (∿) of the respiratory process, the differentiating wave-like form (⌒⌒⌒) of the circulatory process, and the spikey wave-like form (∧∧∧∧) of the nervous system. These rhythms can be sensed by pulses associated with the Chakras.

Listening carefully to systems such as the breathing, heartbeat and brain, one is taken to the center of the Chakra and thence to the spiritual heart as shown in diagram 6.1.

In the diagram you can see the two main flows of conscious energy. One flows from the cosmic heart center through each chakra up towards the higher vibratory rate of spirit. It finds fulfillment in bliss and wisdom with an ever-evolving anticlockwise spiral of love that encompasses and penetrates an ever-increasing vastness of conscious life energy.

The other energy-flow from the cosmic Heart Center is through each Chakra and downward toward the lower vibratory rate of matter. This finds fulfillment in intelligence and action with an involving clockwise spiral of love that manifests and establishes an ever-increasing diversity of life patterns.

Concentration and relaxation are the tools by which consciousness expands and contracts. The universe is expanding and contracting all the time and it is by this natural vibrating motion that energy builds up and interacts with itself to form and experience the common drives (Chakras) that create further forms of life.

When the heart is more tuned to the higher-frequency Chakras of the conceptual, intuitive and imaginative levels, then the consciousness tends to become introverted and looks inward to itself for authority, ideas and visions.

When the heart is more tuned to the lower-frequency Chakras of the intellectual, social and physical levels,

Diagram 6.1.

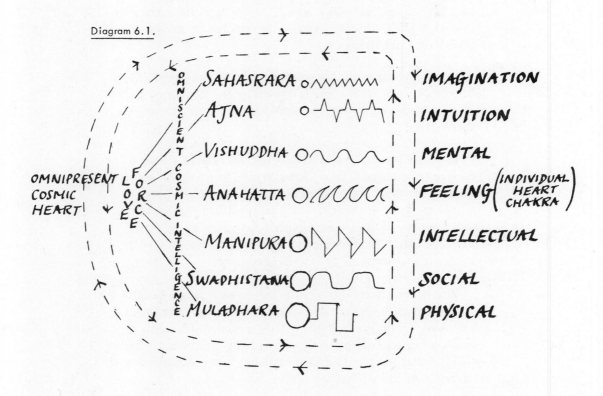

the consciousness tends to become extroverted and looks outward to the environment for knowledge, expansion and sensual contact.

On each level of consciousness, energy builds up logarithmically. Therefore, doubling the effort to grow brings four times the amount of conscious energy expansion.

The mastering of one level, such as the physical level, cannot come totally without some awareness and growth on other levels. Like a house with no owner, a well-developed body is of no spiritual value on its own. In fact, it is difficult to develop a perfect body without awareness of the mind that is moving in it and the one who is consciously caring for it.

It is therefore necessary to be aware of other levels. Growth is more fulfilling when one can move consciousness on any one level and change to any other, with an awareness of the situation of the moment. Some situations call for emphasis on physical action, some for mental alertness and some for spiritual understanding. Some call for a consciousness on all levels. So to be able to move consciousness, firing on all cylinders as it were, is a definite advantage in facing life's challenges and in helping to relate to all beings on all levels as parts of the SELF.

On all levels, we can work inwardly by going into the "nitty gritty" of any deep-seated conditioning and learn how to let go of it by relaxing and seeing the Truth as it is now. We can also work on expansion by concentrating on the Truth as seen anew and from it developing new arts and abilities.

Although there are tendencies toward introversion and extroversion, it is the positive awareness of the whole and the concern for the whole that guides the evolving spiral of life energy back to the source. It is a negative self-indulgence and false identification with the ego that produces a resistance to the life flow and thereby limits consciousness.

Pure consciousness flows eternally from the spiritual heart on all levels and the Source uses both positive and negative aspects of the one energy to relate to a time world.

A knowledge of the flow of electrical energy shows how both positive and negative aspects are contained in the one current flow of energy as positive and negative sides of the circuit. If there were no negativity and resistance to life-flow, the consciousness would short-circuit itself, like shorting out the terminals of a battery. This is sometimes what happens in what is often referred to as a spiritual high. The effect of certain drugs can bring this about suddenly and disastrously. In the true blissful spiritual state of Samadhi, the circuits of the consciousness are highly tuned and the balance of positive to negative and level to level is carefully controlled so that the blissful experience of the source can be manifested in wise action done with direction and with love. This gives a lasting beneficial effect.

Active life energy is called Prana, and passive life energy Apana. In breathing, maximum Prana is experienced at the end of the inhalation and maximum Apana at the end of the exhalation.

With correct breathing, as in the pranayam exercises, Prana and Apana assist one another and life current flows freely, providing that the circuits of the body, mind and soul are in the right state of alignment and attunement.

This state of alignment and attunement can be seen and experienced in:

a) A correctly proportioned body with correct metabolic functioning as developed through the postures of Hatha Yoga.

b) An alert even-mindedness functioning on all levels of consciousness. This can be brought about by breathing excercises and by observation and introspection in practical situations.

c) A peaceful, caring soul that looks at the whole of life with equanimity and understanding. This develops from a study of the laws of consciousness and a willing application of them.

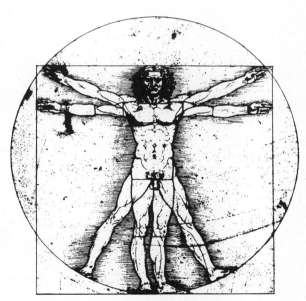

"Study in the proportions of the human body, based on Vitruvius" (1492) by Leonardo da Vinci (1452-1519).

With the above development, the potential difference between positive and negative extremes of life energy is increased. With the power of the will, current flow is a maximum according to the law:

$$\text{Life Current flow (I)} = \frac{\text{Will Power (W)}}{\text{to interest or manifest the SELF}} \Big/ \frac{\text{Potential (V)}}{\substack{\text{to be aware of opportunities and}\\\text{possibilities in life.}}}$$

Will power is dependent upon the individual's capacity to work willingly and to learn with interest and a calm enthusiasm. With R as the resistance to the life energy flow we have a control factor and $W = I^2 R$ and V^2, just the same as in the application of Ohm's law to the flow of electricity through a circuit. The circuit here is life itself and consciousness directs and resists the current flow of energy according to the Will and capacity of the individual.

In terms of balancing the flow of consciousness that may often seem to dart here, there and everywhere, there are basically only four directions the consciousness can go from its center. These are:

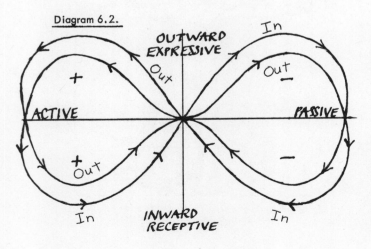

Diagram 6.2.

inwards positive
inwards negative
outwards positive
outwards negative

Inwards and Outwards are relative terms used to indicate the movement of consciousness from its present state, towards either a deeper experience or a fuller expression.

Positive and negative are also relative terms used to denote opposite effects. Positive -- real, dynamic; negative -- illusory passive.

Both positive and negative energy can eventually turn to their opposites. Excessive joy from over stimulation can eventually break into sorrow and in some cases the heart ceases. The consciousness that sees too much sorrow can eventually be moved to seek joy and often finds it in total surrender to God, the greater Self. If there is a continued perseverance in seeking, then each wave of joy and sorrow will be intensified and spiral either towards an expansion of the experience or to an inward refinement of it. With every positive move there is a reflection in its opposite phase. This can be misleading and cause delusion, if the consciousness is lured into false identification with the negative reflection.

However, if there is a constant centering of desires through an inner quietness and a unified relationship with the ONE who is moving consciousness, then each experience will take one to a deeper understanding of consciousness.

On every level of consciousness there are forces of attraction and repulsion. All parts of consciousness, animals, plants, birds, humans, etc., have a magnetic field associated with them. Therefore on every level we may feel an attraction or repulsion towards another person or other part of our whole Self. The attraction may be very strong but not necessarily appropriate to the situation at hand. If it is a positive attraction it will bring an upliftment of consciousness. This means a feeling or sense of recognition of a greater unlimited Self. The consciousness may expand with a sudden feeling of joy, or it may become still and bring an aura of peace to life. The effect can be felt with music, or in a person's voice. It may be seen in certain characteristics in someone's personality, or it may come through the inner sound current of the universe called the AUM vibration. Some people hear an inner voice and realize it to be the God Self.

Both inward and outward positivity increases the life flow and refreshes the experiencer.

Negativity (limiting attitude) produces negative energy which is experienced as a reacting to life energy flow, conflict with others or with the environment and conditions. It is also experienced as disease. The consciousness contracts and resists involvement in life as a whole. There is a feeling of being drained of energy and the result is far from fulfilling.

The completion of a positive cycle of effort produces a positive cycle of events which leads to a greater understanding of life, an expansion of abilities and a release of "karma".

Karma is the law of cause and effect; of action and reaction. Consciousness goes where we put it and if we can see the effects which we produce by our actions upon others and upon other areas of our own life, then we see what will be reflected back at us by the life process.

If, when we move consciousness, we leave gaps in the form of remorse or hidden desires, then those gaps will cause a psychic vaccum which nature abhors and so has to fill. Similarly, if there is an urge to control without the ability to do so, then any resentments or suppressions in the consciousness will produce psychic pressures which will have to be released --- hence Karma!

Karmic patterns are built up whenever there is a reaction to action. Duality separates and identification with the separateness brings attachment to it. The law of Karma is life's way of reflecting back to the SELF, the state of affairs. Attachment and false identification bring pain and suffering.

Tracing actions, thoughts and feelings back to their source by asking oneself "Why is this so?" and investigating thoroughly, is a way of understanding one's own Karmic patterns. Objective analysis frees one from identification. The ability to accept life as it is and to surrender to actions that reflect Truth frees one from suffering.

With awareness we have the potential to change.
With will power we have the ability to change.
With attunement — waiting for the right time, place and state of consciousness — that change of energy can bring benefit to the whole of consciousness, and at the same time release one from the Law of Karma.

The balancing of expression and receptivity to Truth, which is the subject of this part of the course, is another way of finding release from Karma.

Whenever there is stillness, which is the result of the balance of energies, there is the opportunity to observe objectively that which is moving and thereby see the True situation.

Another way is to learn the art of relaxation to the extent of releasing all actions, thoughts and feelings, etc., from the conscious state. Certain techniques that produce trance states can enable one to do this temporarily. However, techniques alone are not able to provide total release from Karma. The reason for Karma has to be understood before the will to release it can be effective. Enlightenment comes before liberation and the need to become enlightened has to be felt before effort can be made. In the effort applied, law is understood and the clarity grows to prepare the way for total enlightenment. This provides the higher consciousness that can handle the responsibility that enlightenment brings. It is the wise use of this responsibility and the love of freedom that gives rise to the final liberation from Karmic influence.

Being uninfluenced by all conscious events yet responsible for their fulfillment, one IS IN TRUTH IN THE ONE.

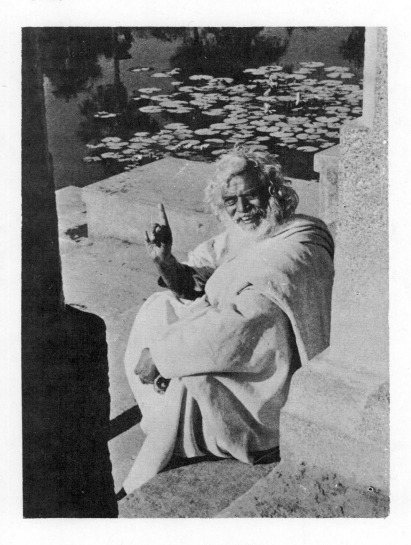

DAILY PRACTICE FOR PART 6

THEME: *SEE WITH THE SOUL THAT*
SEES ITS OWN ESSENCE
HEAR WITH THE HEART THAT
BEATS ITS OWN SILENCE

The human body is made up of many parts; the part is part of the whole universe. An arm or a leg has its special functions and characteristics but it cannot operate except as part of the whole body. Just so with the individual consciousness: "individual" means "undividable". Therefore the individual is a part of the One, and each aspect of that individuality (male/female, positive/negative, light/dark) is an aspect of the One. So if your consciousness can embrace All, you can realize that there is no separation between a selfish self and others, or between Selfless Self and THE SELF. The ego qualifies and labels, and causes an illusion of separation. The centered state of being is one without delusions.

POSTURE PRACTICE

The routine of postures at the beginning of Section 1 gives a balanced order of pose and counterpose --- e.g. standing inverted; inverted Backbend and Twist; Backbend and Twist/sitting forward bending/lying and sitting.

For each type of posture there is also a Shiva/Shakti balance. Shiva postures are those that enhance the male qualities --- aspiring, creative, energizing, uplifting, etc. Shakti postures are those that enhance the female qualities --- receptive, sensitive, calming, passive, etc. In the routine given, notice this Shiva/Shakti balance between Headstand/Shoulderstand, Dhanurasana/Chakrasana, upright Spinal Twist/lying down Spinal Twist.

Male and Female are aspects of Polarity which is relative and therefore variable in as much as one posture may be more female than another, but it can still be male with respect to another. For example, Forward Bending in the sitting position generally increases Shakti energy. However, with respect to lying down (Savasana) and Yoga Mudra it is more male. Standing postures definitely increase the Shiva energy yet Uttanasana is encouraging a more receptive nature than, for instance, the Warrior Pose

133

which is a very firm posture. The Shoulderstand which is female compared to the Headstand is itself male compared to the Plow.

The important feature of Pose/Counterpose -- Shiva/Shakti postures is to sense within the balancing effect and to recognize what is experienced in the consciousness when you are in the state of balance.

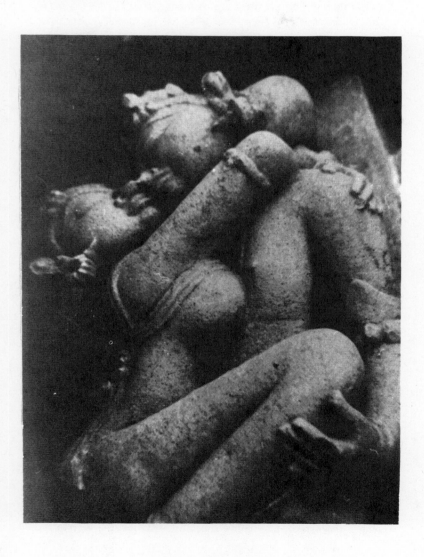

PRANAYAM: HEALTH THROUGH BREATH
THE BALANCING BREATH
(ALTERNATE NOSTRIL BREATHING)

1) Sit in the upright position with the shoulders well back. Extend the neck and drop the head onto the chest, at the same time raising the sternum to meet it. This locks the throat in what is called Jalabandha (a bandha is a lock which creates a partial vacuum).

2) Bend the index and forefinger of the right hand forwards into the palm and hold in position with the thumb mound.

3) Place the tip of the thumb lightly on the right side of the nose, just below the nose-bone. Place the tip of the fourth and fifth fingers on the left side of the nose with the fourth finger up also next to the nose-bone and the little finger resting against the outer edge of the nostril.

4) Close the right nostril by putting the thumb against the bone in the nose and inhale for seven beats up the left nostril, controlling the inflow by light pressure from the fourth and fifth fingers against the nose-bone and flange of the left nostril.

5) Close both nostrils by placing the fourth finger against the bone fully and holding the breath for a count of three beats.

6) Lift the thumb away and exhale through the right nostril for seven beats, controlling the outflow by careful positioning of the tip of the thumb against the nose-bone.

7) Now take the breath up the right nostril for seven beats.

8) Close and hold for three beats.

9) Remove the third and fourth fingers and exhale through the left nostril for seven beats.

Repeat this complete cycle about twelve times.

FURTHER PRACTICE

After doing the above exercise for three months, change the ratio of inhalation/hold/exhalation from 7:3:7 to 8:8:8 and increase to 8:16:8 after a further three months.

135

APPLICATION TO LIFE

Try going about your work without using the pronoun "I". Attribute what is done to the fact that it is done without a personal qualification. In relationships, look at what is said and done, but see it from the viewpoint of and interaction between the fields of feeling consciousness and the body consciousness through which energy is being transferred. In other words, be impersonal for a time in order to experience the timeless dimension operating in a time-space continuum, and see how ALL IS ONE; THE ONE WATCHES ALL.

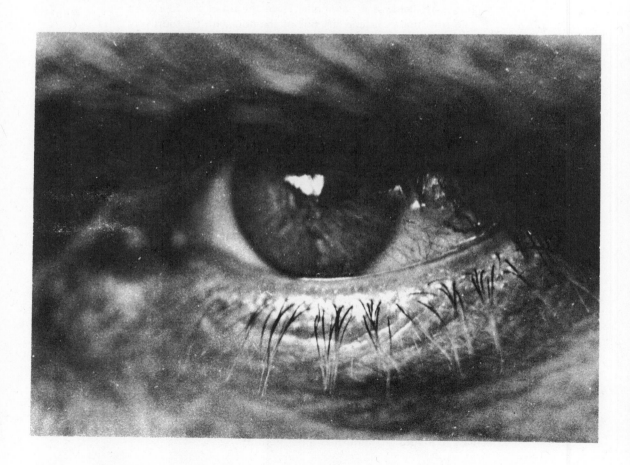

PART 7

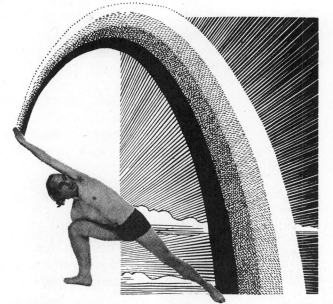

RELATING BODY TO LEVELS OF VIBRATION AND COLOR

PRACTICAL SITUATION --- SELF MOTIVATION

An emotion is an energy of motion (e-motion) which we all have and can develop for good use. As long as we are using the emotions and they are not using us, then we have the freedom to experience and express through this vibration. In the mapping of consciousness emotions lie between the green heart-feeling and the blue throat-authority level.

The color of the emotional vibration is a greenish-blue, and emotional tensions and flexibility are indicated in the shoulders. Psychologically we can experience how centered we are on the emotional level in the following ways.

1) Note your response to T.V. programs, books, the drama of life's events, and arts such as music and painting. What is it that most stirs your emotions to want to do something, to experience something or to express something, in your way?

    Can you see which areas drain you of energy, giving you "the blues"? Perhaps the ill treatment of certain sections of humanity or perhaps a certain type of music brings tears to your eyes through association. If you are affected negatively by these emotions, pratice facing them in a more objective, intellectual way. Look for the cause in yourself and see how you can "let them go". Know that there is always a good reason for things when you can see the whole picture.

    Can you see which areas are positive for you, uplifting you with energy, giving you the expansion of "blue skies"? Practice using this energy for devotion to the ONE who created the opportunity to experience this area of life that gives you uplift-ment. Devotion is a blue level emotional type of energy which can be manifested as actions, words, a furthering of a worthy cause, or simply a giving of pure being in terms of a sincere "thank you".

2) If you have a friend or group to do these exercises with, test each other's emotional response by seeing how "straight" you can be in the face of the other person:

> laughing at you,
> crying before you.

Change places and express:
> lamentation,
> disgust of any negativity you can see.

Make erotic gestures in front of each other and chant or sing love songs to each other. Give praise and show devotion to the highest in each other. Remember that you are expressing and experiencing the above underlined emotional patterns.

Self-motivation on the conceptual level can be seen by answering the following questions in writing or verbally.

"How do you experience being centered, or feeling the presence of God?"

"How do you experience being told what to do? Do you mind or react?"

"How do you use your own authority to communicate to another person what has to be done?"

The blue level is the level of memory and authority. The center of the blue level is experienced in harmony, peace, expansion and devotion. How close to the center of the blue level do you think you come?

STUDY MATERIAL

THE BODY IS A MAP OF CONSCIOUSNESS

Energy expands and contracts according to the nature of the motivating force behind it. Heat and pressure cause a change in vibration. Such is the case when ice is melted by heat into water and evaporated into steam. Pressure condenses it back from the rarefied state into the solid form. However, in the process a purification has taken place and can be seen by the falling away of the dirt particles and the reformation of the pure water particles.

The purification of consciousness by internal heat and pressure changes the vibration. The movement of energy and the change in its vibration is reflected on all levels. On the body level shape, form and quality of reproduction from the internal original can be seen. We can see how bulges in the physical form are the manifestations of the shaping of the mind which in turn is developed from the subtler depths of consciousness.

Without desire or the urge to express, consciousness is like a straight line, an unmodulated direct current of energy, or a universe of emptiness. Without desire or urge, the body would be like a hollow tube, with an inner core of emptiness and an outer shell of evenly distributed matter. It is interesting to note that there is in fact more space in the atoms of the body than there is matter. As soon as some urge or desire is put into consciousness, then content and contour lines indicate the direction and flow of consciousness from stillness to some new level of consciousness. For inner stillness to be maintained there is a need for the balance of energy on that level; a readjustment of urges and desires. Desire and urge can take the consciousness on a whole experiential trip, through always seeking newness, balance and a return to the original state of stillness.

This is the journey of life and the body can be our map as we explore the avenues through which our consciousness has traveled. The direction in which it is at present moving and the route we need to take in quest of the peace from knowing the SELF is the benefit of this study of body-map reading.

When energy is released from the nucleus of the body cells, it expands and contracts in such a way that an expansion creates an inner pressure and pushes out the walls of the cells and hence the outer body. This energy pattern may form either a shapely bulge when controlled, or excessive fatness when it is out of control. A contraction of the body cells causes the body to cave inward and this may be seen as either an attractive waistline in the body structure when there is awareness or a "wasting away" when there is too much rigidity.

In bringing the omnipresent state of pure consciousness into perfect manifestation it is dimensionalized in the body. Around the center line of the body, energy is distributed according to the nature of the consciousness forming it.

The *front* of the body shows the nature of the outgoing expressive energies.

The *back* of the body shows the inward introspective state of affairs.

The *right side* of the body shows the nature of the male reasoning aspects.

The *left side* of the body shows the nature of the female feeling aspects.

The *top* of the body shows the nature of the spiritual aspirations.

The *lower half* of the body shows the nature of the physical manifestation.

141

The balancing of the above energies and the correct proportioning of the body parts makes for a perfect body. Attunement with the SELF within and with all aspects of life encourages this heaven on earth and brings about realization of the wholeness of life. Any out-of-attunement or imbalance is shown in the body, so that the SELF may see itself and reshape the energies into a true reflection of the SELF.

From diagram 7.1 you will see that areas of the body show the manifestation of associated psychological and spiritual drives. As the material state of consciousness is brought to the stature of the spiritual SELF, the spirit of the absolute descends into matter to describe itself through matter. There is an interplay of self-expression and self-reflection. Interactions of these cause heat and a fusing into the solid form. Separations cause freezing and a disintegration of the solid form. Hence we see in old age a hardening of the skin with contractions and deep crevices in the skin. In the new born babe we see a softness and suppleness in the skin. Look at yourself in a mirror and feel the texture of your skin. Note where energy is projecting and where there is a lack.

The front of the body shows what type of energy is being expressed and to what extent. It shows our conscious nature. Where the energy is concentrated, there is an emphasis on a particular level. For example, a large chest shows an emphasis of the security level, a big heart and a giving of nourishment. Women are naturally inclined to an emphasis of this level in order to nourish God's children. Energy in the stomach shows an expression of the intellect and a concern for social activity. There could be several effects of this, from the teaching of a compassionate Buddha to a man who likes his drink with the guys at the bar. Energy in the front of the legs shows physical possibilities and reproductive virility. Pronounced facial features such as bumps on the forehead and the forehead sloping back give indication of

142

intuitive and imaginative abilities. A broad face gives a broad outlook on things.

Remember that pure energy can take on any shape. It is the will and awareness that motivate it and give it structure, form and stature. The consciousness may express for selfish reasons or as a selfless act of love. A fat stomach may mean an intellect full of knowledge or a belly full of food. In either case it is the way it is used and balanced with the rest of consciousness that determines its relevance to the center and Truth.

The back of the body shows what type of energy is being experienced. It shows our unconscious nature. In cases of over-emphasis, this needs to be expressed. For example, arched shoulders and protruding dorsal show too much inward emotion. This needs to be expressed by lifting up the heart and channelling the energy into other areas, by positive physial action perhaps. This will help in the correct reshaping of the body and of consciousness as a whole. A broad back shows an inward expanse of mind energies. Large hips and buttocks can result from an excess of physical urges or indulgences.

All energies can be rechannelled. A look at the contour of the front and back of your body can show possible directions for the flow to take, so that an evenness and balance of the areas between the center to front of the body and center to back of the body is achieved.

The right side of the body shows how energy is expressed. This is the male, active, giving, assertive side. A flexibility in the right shoulder shows flexibility in emotional activity. A strong right arm is a powerful tool for acting our feelings. Emphasis on the right side when walking indicates assertive and possible dominating inclinations.

The left side of the body shows how energy is experienced. This is the female, passive, receptive, sensitive side. Flexibility in the left shoulder shows emotional adaptability. An emphasis on the left side when walking can show a tendency to lean on the female qualities of one's nature.

Emphasis on the outer edges of the body (shown by soles of shoes) shows tendencies to extroversion. Introversion is indicated by turned-in knees and emphasis on the inner soles of the feet.

An imbalance of left to right energies (male to female relationship within oneself) will be seen by an uneven penetration through the eyes. Alternate nostril breathing given in the daily practice which follows brings about a balance in the male and female aspects of the consciousness.

The height of the body shows why we express ourselves in the way that we do. A tall body shows an aspiring, reaching-up character. When the consciousness is drooping, so does the body and especially the heart. A tall body is often a thin body because of individual refinement and concern for Spiritual values.

The shortness of the body shows why we experience the way we do. A stocky body is often full of joy and down to earth. A short plump person is often ambitious in the world and radiates outwards to it.

If you have a straight character your body will display that straightness. A curvacious body shows an artistic nature. If you are cautious you will probably walk mainly on your toes. If you are firm in your decisions your heel will come down firmly on the ground well before the toes. A right foot pointing outwards affirms established values. If you stand with the left foot outwards, somewhere in your consciousness is the desire to point out your feelings.

The texture of the skin gives a clue as to who is motivating, expressing and experiencing through it. Hard, soft, rough or smooth skin is created by the nature of the person within. A thick skinned person finds stability in earthly-type qualities and physical realities. "Skinny" people have their consciousness "nearer to the bone" where soul type qualities and mental concepts are more of a reality. Watery skin indicates maternal tendencies, dry skin shows paternal tendencies.

Thin and wiry, short and fat, all shapes and skin textures are the result of moving consciousness, either consciously or unconsciously. Change the shape of the body, and the one within is re-mind-ed of the change by the sense of new positioning and the associated change in the mind and other layers of consciousness. The way the change takes place comes from the nature of the person and reflects in the condition of the body.

Hence it is possible to look at ourself; to look at our own state of consciousness and at our nature, since problems in each area of consciousness will reflect in the body and will show up in the appropriate place. For example, a doubting of one's ability to reason and to know (male aspect) causes negativity in the intellect. This will show in the right side of the abdomen either internally or externally according to one's introverted or extroverted tendencies.

Although it is possible to work out problems through yoga postures, it is also helpful to be able to also work consciously on the psychological level and in all cases look deeper and deeper at the cause of defect since the defect will occur again and again until the cause has been seen and eliminated. An effective technique for looking at the causes is Creative Conflict*. Since most

* Creative Conflict is a copyright name. See "The Rise of the Phoenix: Universal Government by Nature's Laws" (See Booklist).

145

of our problems arise from causes that are buried in our unconscious, the process of Creative Conflict uses a group of people to skillfully probe the hidden depths of our nature and help bring about a permanent change in our being.

Use the information above to understand the cause of any tensions and the shaping of your own body and then work on as many places of development as you can.

A falling left side means a falling of the female nature. See if it originates in the legs, body or neck. When you have located the area of the source of the deformity, see if you can find the cause. Even physical accidents can be the karmic effect of a cause which indicates disharmony with nature and which may still be a pattern in the consciousness. Look for faulty mental and spiritual behavior.

Lift the left side from the point where it is falling and concentrate on keeping it in position. In time it could become even with the other side. Look for any conflict reflected inwards by the repositioning. If the cause is an old mental pattern it can be seen when you are trying to counteract it with a change in posture.

Remember that correct proportions and a still even gaze through the eyes are an indication of balance. Tall, short, thin and fat are relative conditions and have to be considered in relation to the situation and circumstances. If there is a deficiency such as a limb or organ missing, do the best you can with what is available and emphasize the function of the missing part in other ways. For example -- no right arm - assertive action.

As awareness increases it is very easy to start assessing and judging the faults and deformities of others. Remember that what we see is only a reflection of ourself. If the self is judging, look at why. We can only see the reality of another person's consciousness to the extent that we can see our own. If you want to learn from others, look for the cause of both the radiance shining through the eyes of a soul filled with goodness and of a soul empty through negativity. Look for the person with control and flexibility used for the benefit of others as well as seeing the lazy bones who is self indulgent. Look for the joy that bubbles spontaneously and the love that is given unconditionally, as well as seeing the ego that seeks only for its own ends. Then look at the attitude to life and the lifestyle of the one who reflects all things.

Observe, experience, give where the need is calling, but be guided by the wisdom that sees which need is the most important and relevant. All states of illness, disease, addiction and corruption are the effects of delusion. We don't have to agree with them or identify with them but we cannot ignore them. It is by them that we can learn to understand the need for them and how to eliminate them as we grow and expand to know and acknowledge more fully the ONE SELF. In acquiring the skill in moving consciousness in the way that spirit and nature intended - with awareness and a pure heart, then we evolve more and more towards a heaven on earth.

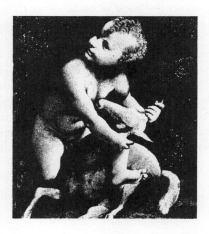

DAILY PRACTICE FOR PART 7

THEME: *WHAT IS NATURAL*
WHAT IS CONDITIONAL
WHAT IS HABITUAL
WHAT IS ESSENTIAL

Notice what is natural and what is unnatural. What may seem to be natural may be a comfortable habit and not valid in the present situation. Fashions in clothes, eating and living often restrict correct breathing and encourage bad habits in posture, metabolic balance and mental attitudes.

Look at the effects of all that you do, think and feel. Experiment with what you learn in this course. Discriminate and check with honest feedback from true friends and life itself. Consciousness sees only what is of itself. See what nature is playing back to you. Is it your song? Is it the song celestial?

POSTURE PRACTICE --- PRANA AND APANA

Postures which open up the chest and extend the front of the body increase the positive (manifested) currents of energy in the body when correctly co-ordinated with the inhalation of the breath.

Postures which contract the abdominal area and draw the consciousness inwards increase the negative (unmanifested) currents of energy in the body when correctly co-ordinated with the exhalation of the breath.

Remember that both excitation and stillness are necessary for the flow of energy. As in the flow of electricity, there has to be a positive and a negative pole for there to be a potential difference and hence an attracting power which draws the currents of energy around the circuit. In the context above, positive currents emphasize motion, activity and an outgoing viewpoint. Negative currents emphasize stillness, passivity and an ingoing viewpoint.

When the Prana and Apana are balanced and increased by co-ordinating posture with breathing, then provided there is an ease of motion (little resistance to movement), the power of the consciousness will also increase.

Power = Current of Energy X Potential Difference

Conscious Ability = Smooth Breathing X Prana: Apana in Posture Movement

INCREASING PRANA

Stand upright in Tadasana. Inhale for eight beats while raising the arms in front of you and above the head. Hold for eight beats. Exhale for eight beats lowering the arms. Repeat with counts of 10.10.10, then 12.12.12, and then 10.10.10, and back to 8.8.8.

INCREASING APANA

Lie down with the back on the floor. Inhale for six beats and on the exhalation, bend the knees and bring them up to the chest to a count of six beats. Hold the breath out for six beats. Inhale for six beats, taking the arms over the head and returning the legs to the ground. Repeat, bringing legs up to chest for eight beats, holding breath out for eight beats and then inhaling and stretching legs and arms for eight beats. Continue with counts of 10.10. 10, 8.8.8., and finally 6.6.6.

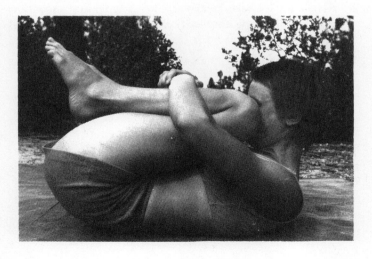

COMBINED PRANA/APANA BALANCE

UTTANASANA:

Standing upright in Tadasana,

1) Inhale for eight beats raising the arms forwards and above the head.

2) Hold for four beats with the arms outstretched behind the ears. Look at the fingertips.

3) Exhale for eight beats and reach well forward to bring the arms to the ground. Bend from the waist and keep the tail bone well up and the spine straight, also keeping the legs straight, the arms straight and well behind the ears, and the feet flat on the ground.

4) Hold out for four beats with head, shoulders and arms relaxed.

5) Inhale for eight beats, coming up to the standing position with the head leading and the arms completely relaxed and hanging loosely by the sides. Exhale for eight beats.

6) Repeat the above three to six times.

UKTANASANA:

Stand upright in Tadasana and exhale completely.

1) Inhale for six beats while raising the arms sideways above the head and behind the ears, palms facing each other.

2) Exhale for six beats bending the knees to take up a squatting position. Have the arms well behind the ears and the feet flat on the floor.

3) Inhale and come up to a count of six beats straightening the legs and body.

4) Exhale bringing the arms down to the side of the body to a count of six beats.

5) Repeat three to six times.

Lie down on the back and breathe smoothly and evenly. Examine the state of the consciousness.

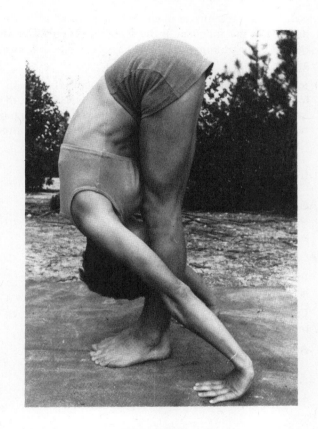

UTTANASANA

PRANAYAM --- HEALTH THROUGH BREATH
CLEANSING BREATHS

STAGE 1 -- HA AND HER BREATHS

1) Kneel in Vajrasana or sit on a chair. Let the palms of the hands face downwards on the knees.

   Inhale fully with the mouth closed.

   Exhale with the mouth open, speaking the syllable HA and drawing in the abdomen at the same time. Using suggestion, rid the body of impurities from lower to upper parts as you exhale.

2) Inhale again with the mouth closed and exhale with the mouth open, this time speaking the syllable HER and thrusting the tongue out as the abdomen is drawn in. Using suggestion, rid the body of impurities from the outside extremes (shoulders, ribs, etc.) as you exhale.

3) Repeat HA and HER breaths five times.

STAGE 2 -- NORMAL BREATHS

Take three Normal Breaths.

STAGE 3 -- BELLOWS BREATH

Inhale through the nostrils letting breath push out the abdomen at the front.

Exhale through the nostrils pushing the breath out by the quick drawing inwards of the abdomen.

Repeat 10 times.

STAGE 4 -- ENERGIZING BREATHS

Take three Energizing Breaths to a count of 10.

Repeat stages 1 to 3 a total of three times.

APPLICATION TO LIFE

Having learned how to build up power, learn also how to use it wisely in sharing it with others. Examine what communication means in terms of relating and sharing energy with others. When you see someone doing other than what you think they "ought" to do or "should" do, look at what you are seeing and at what that judgement is reflecting in yourself. If you see what you perceive as shortcomings in another person, try to communicate it to him, not by telling him what to do, but rather by seeing the need and encouraging the good qualities in both yourself and the other person. Then the *real* need will be fulfilled, and with a deeper understanding of the Oneness.

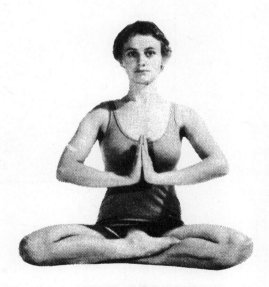

PERFECT POSE

The diagram below shows the variations from the unmodified state of a straight tube to a body shaped to provide the most effective functioning and natural expression.

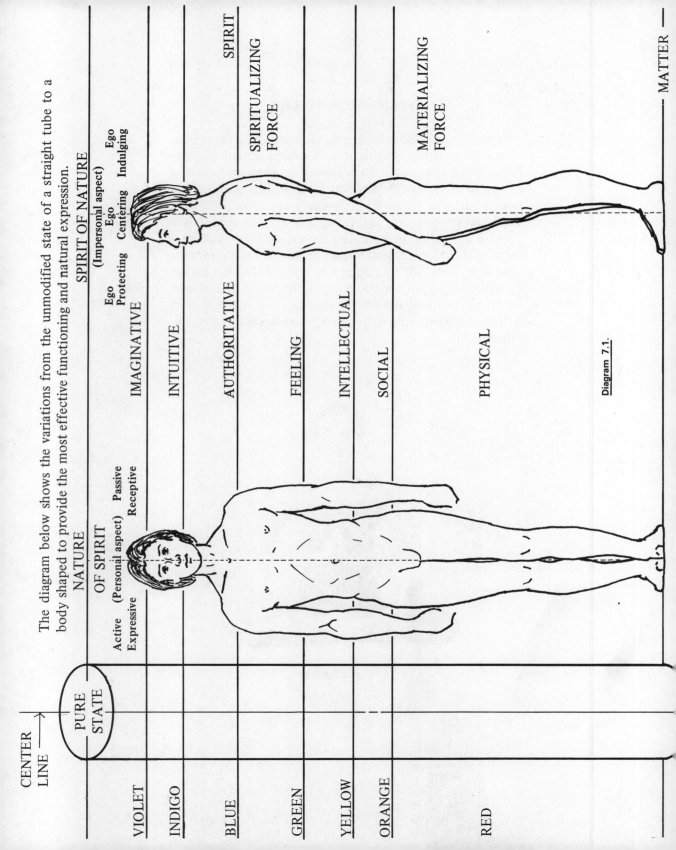

Diagram 7.1.

PART 8

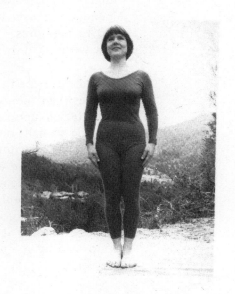

THE COMPLETE PERSON AND THE NUCLEAR DRIVES

PRACTICAL SITUATION -- INTUITIVE KNOWING

One way of knowing something is by the use of the intuition. The reasoning and logic of the intellect, the thinking mind and feeling heart are all valid ways through which to experience knowing, but they do very often depend upon past information, conditioning and comparative measures. With the intuition we learn how to know without knowing why we know.

The center for the intuition is the center of the forehead between the eyes. Start this practical session with a meditation upon that center. Sit comfortably with the spine straight and the hands resting on the lap with the palms facing upwards. Relax by watching the breath and then turn the eyes upwards to the center, behind the forehead. Become very still, relaxed but very attentive and look deeply into this center of the intuition. If you see any colors or a circle of light shining in the darkness, observe it and acknowledge it, but don't be hypnotized by it. Keep the wakefulness of an attentive observer.

It is at this point that you can ask a question and receive a direct answer to it. You can ask something about yourself, such as what is it that you need to know right now for further enlightenment, or you can ask a question about the past or future. If you put a concern about another person to the intuition you may see directly what it is that could help him.

When you ask a question, wait for an answer but don't expect or assume the answer. Time delays are sometimes experienced, but usually the first flash is the intuitive answer. Intuitive knowing depends upon a certain confidence that the right answer will come if it is right to come and when it is right to come. Be relaxed and be attentive. Assume the attitude you would when asking someone his name: you do not anticipate an answer, but merely wait for a response.

In this way you can find out relevant information about yourself and about others; about lost articles, lost information, future events, future needs.

You can also do this with a friend and practice the intuiting of each other's thoughts as in telepathy. You can also find out each other's main drive. An extension of this is in the use of the pendulum, where the pendulum acts as an extension of the psychic nervous system and can be trained to swing according to a YES/NO answering technique. Simple experiments and step-by-step instructions in this art can be found in *Alive to the Universe*. The most complete book available on the subject is *Supersensonics* (see book list).

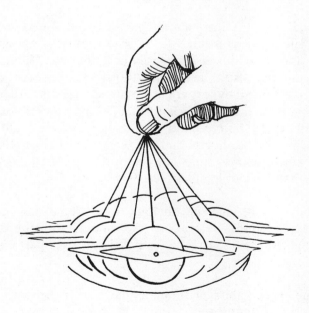

STUDY MATERIAL

SUMMARY OF SECTION 2

In section two we have been dealing with the mechanics of the mind and the evolution of consciousness through a knowledge of the various levels of consciousness as set out by Christopher Hills in *Nuclear Evolution: Discovery of the Rainbow Body.*.

Please note that with all techniques, your intentions must be pure in order for them to bear fruit. If there is any I, me or limiting self in the way of the direct flow from the Source, then the answers will be relevant only to that state of consciousness, and untruths will come as well as truths. Be centered in the wholeness of things and what appears will be relevant to that wholeness in you.

What we put into consciousness is seen with consciousness and continues to be seen until it is removed from the conscious or subconscious levels. Act, think or feel and the results are seen. Repeat the process and it is reinforced by experience and association. Repeat a third time and a habit is formed. This process works on all levels, body, mind and soul. The "I" that is conscious of the habits that are formed in the conscious and subconscious minds has the opportunity to change if the habit is causing ill effect.

Some habits may be obvious to us; some may not. Certain patterns of routine movement, thought and feeling are necessary for survival in our particular environment.

There are habits of thought that lead to frustration, confusion or depression, simply because they rely upon others for their fulfillment. Unless checked, this reliance upon others can lead to demand and imposition upon their freedom.

To change, we need flexibility; to hold fast to that which is true, we need firmness. Will power is a great tool for evolution if it can be used wisely. The ability to surrender to the flow of life current is an asset if it is done with pure love. To be in full control one needs to be in constant contact with the still center within; nonattached to the worldly life but able to move the consciousness in it.

When by observation and practice one can see and guide which way the consciousness is moving, then one can assist the balance of nature accordingly. Too much firmness brings rigidity, tension and pain. Too much flexibility brings looseness, laziness and suffering. At any one time there is a combination of assisting and resisting flows of energy which together bring about both the ease of flow required for flexibility and the control of flow required for firmness.

When these energies are realized and guided with awareness, concentration and relaxation, a new balance of energies can be experienced. This applies to the Reverse Triangle posture in the following way. Firmness is required first in the feet and legs. Remember to relax before stretching and positioning any part. Holding the feet and legs firm, it is next important to have flexibility of movement in the pelvic area, so that one side of the sacrum can drop toward the floor, and the other side can lift up toward the ceiling. This movement assists in the perfect positioning of the body. Without this movement there is a resistance to the correct positioning. Once in position, firmness needs to be brought into the pelvic area while the trunk of the body is made flexible in order to extend fully forward.

Eventually, the whole posture is held firm in the shape while the mind is relaxed and made flexible enough to examine each part of the body and the whole of it in more detail.

As the consciousness goes deeper, the mind is held firm and flexibility moves to the soul level while subtler currents of energy in the body and mind are examined.

In this way, firmness and flexibility are motivated and balanced from deeper and deeper levels and an evolutionary step to a "heightened" or tuned expression of consciousness is made. The degree of this evolutionary effort is shown in the perfect dimensions of the posture, the correct proportioning of the body, the mindfulness and the ease with which every centimeter of the body is made conscious.

The same consciousness that is becoming more aware through posture and movement can be developed on other levels of consciousness by the same approach.

On every level of consciousness a subtle magnetic field of energy emanates with an attracting assisting force and repelling resisting force inherent in it. We can experience this on each level in daily life. An attraction on the physical level may be to have physical contact or sexual relations with another person. On the mental level it may be the desire to share ideas. On the spiritual level it may be a need to meditate with a group or to follow a particular guru. Similarly we may be repelled by all these. What makes the attraction and repulsion valid is the situation and the state of consciousness in which they are experienced. If there is a willingness to explore Truth and change accordingly, then positive attraction will bring upliftment to the consciousness. This means a feeling or sense of recognition of the unlimited higher Self. The consciousness expands and one may feel an indescribable joy, or one may become still and feel at peace with life. Both female (inward) and male (outward) positivity increases the life energy flow and refreshes the consciousness. Negative life energy is experienced as a resistance to life flow, conflict with others, the environment or conditions, and as disease within one's own body. Examples of the male (expansion) and the female (contraction) aspects of consciousness expressing and experiencing positively and negatively on each level are shown on following pages.

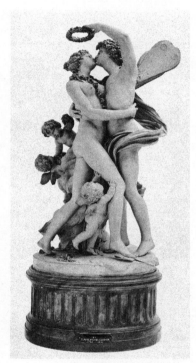

Frick Collection, N.Y.

Clodion, Cupid and Psyche

EXPANSION (MALE)

DRIVE	POSITIVE	NEGATIVE
SENSES	Pro-creation and recreation on the physical plane is an act of worship, gratitude to, or glorification of, the true life spirit.	Act of pro-creation is a self-indulgence and physical work is done selfishly.
SOCIAL	Social interaction is for the common good.	Self-esteem is the motivation for social gathering.
INTELLEC-TUAL	Through reason and logic one acknowledges a cosmic intelligence that is guiding all things.	The questioning mind is closed to answers coming from outside of existing knowledge and experience.
SECURITY	An equal love for all beings is the motivating force of action and all things are acquired in order to give to others.	Love is limited to those things that bring personal security.
AUTHORITY	The worship of Truth and peace is the motivating force by which one lives.	Outward authority is followed blindly and a "Comfortable" peace that neglects facing the Truth is allowed to thrive.
INTUITION	Ideals that encompass all beings are sought and manifested.	The future is dreamed of and ideas seen, but are not materialized for others to share.
IMAGI-NATION	Descriptions of reality are expressed in a creative form that causes others to look at the nature of their essential being.	One lives in a dream world of utopia, out of touch with the reality of things and the real needs of others here and now.

CONTRACTION (FEMALE)

DRIVE	POSITIVE	NEGATIVE
SENSES	Producing and nurturing the physical needs of others with a love that supports a creative use of the life energy.	Actions and physical nurturing is for sensuous and self-rewarding purposes only.
SOCIAL	One is ever ready to listen to those who seek help.	One meets others only for self gain.
INTELLEC-TUAL	The cosmic intelligence with the answers to all problems is sought humbly within oneself.	Consciousness is limited by human reasoning based only on a series of sequential facts.
SECURITY	The desire for security takes one inwards to the source of life and makes one less dependent upon others for material nourishment.	Possessions are sought for personal security and satisfaction.
AUTHORITY	Devotion is given to Truth as seen in oneself.	Devotion is given to seeking self-satisfaction in terms of "nice" feelings rather than true fulfillment.
INTUITION	The source is sought within oneself through meditation, listening and direct knowing.	There is a desire to sit in meditation as an escape from worldly duties, or when mechanical thinking gives precedence over inventiveness and true learning.
IMAGI-NATION	There is an inner search for absolute existence which is complete and in all things.	Inner scenes and fantasies take one away from the search for one's true existence.

Observing, experiencing, discriminating and acting with concern for the reality of the moment is the way to intelligent living. Acknowledging the presence of a Unifying Principle and seeing by direct perception is the way to wisdom.

We may learn from what has gone before and predict the future from a series of events. The intellect can do this well. The imagination can support those predictions and dream up a world around them. With the inner stillness the intuition can guide us into unknown realms and with right thinking and feeling we can be motivated into right action in any situation not only for ourself but also for society's benefit.

To understand the energy patterns of each of the seven levels, it is important to learn what it is on each level that motivates positivity and what it is that negates that which is true.* Study the levels in yourself and in others by observing, noting your own reactions to actions, words, thoughts and feelings, etc. Relate them to what is true and what is not true in terms of what is passing and what is permanent.

Remember that consciousness in its pure state is not of the mind and therefore does not mind what it sees. It does not forcefully act and therefore does not react to what it experiences. Pure consciousness is present everywhere and that everywhere is nowhere when, in that pure state, we can free the self from identification with time and space. It is the identification with time and space that causes movement and it is the identification with movement that causes attachment and hence the illusion that the world alone is the reality of life. This is the cause of suffering --- ignorance of our immortal nature.

* There are many interviews with people on different levels of consciousness in "Nuclear Evolution: Discovery of the Rainbow Body" pages 235-345. See Booklist.

The spiritual life is one of retracing our steps back to the non-identified state of the Self under the guidance of the all-seeing source. When the Self sees all as itself and the consciousness becomes pure, there is no need or desire for attachment to any one thing.

In this pure state, evolution is a willingness to change and to see things anew; to find joy in a love of self-giving and receiving without separation between the giver, receiver and that which is given and received. In this oneness with the all-pervading life force is the direct perception of Truth, the reality of life.

The realization of the true Self can come in a flash or be discovered by a steady development in seeing with direct perception. So far we have looked and listened. This is all part of the development. In the next section we will look beyond the mind and to the ways of meditation for the seeing power of direct perception and for the power of love in pure consciousness.

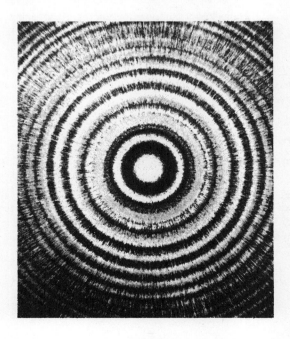

DAILY PRACTICE FOR PART 8

THEME:
WHEN THE CONSCIOUSNESS IS STILL,
THE SELF CAN BE REALIZED
WHEN THE CONSCIOUSNESS IS MOVED,
THE SELF CAN BE SEEN

In yoga, stillness and movement are combined through the simultaneous collaboration of a disciplined intelligence and a spontaneous freedom in the "now".

POSTURE PRACTICE -- SUMMARY

One can do a posture with the male, assertive aspect, or one can see a posture as being done with the female, sensitive aspect. Some postures emphasize the male aspect of consciousness (Shiva) and some postures emphasize the female aspect (Shakti). The aim of yoga is to balance these energies so that there is no conflict of separation to cause a tension or a resistance to movement.

GENERALLY

Standing and backbending postures increase the prana --- the active, dynamic life energies --- and therefore encourage the male aspect.

Inverted and forward bending postures increase the apana --- the passive quietening life energies --- and therefore encourage the female aspect.

Twisting postures help to combine the two aspects

Balancing postures help to stabilize the two aspects.

Lying down postures help to bring the consciousness to rest.

In the center between doing something and letting it be done is the indefinable composite state in which stillness, balance, and activity in a passive manner are all seen as one. This is the meditative state that is to be sought at all times, in every posture, every movement, and in every breath.

166

AS A GUIDELINE

Inhale when the body is opening up at the front to increase Prana naturally.

Exhale when the body is closing up at the front to increase the Apana naturally.

Stretch always on the exhalation. The exception to this rule is the natural stretch on the inhalation when the body needs extra energizing such as the stretch when one first arises from sleep.

On the inhalation observe objectively.

On the exhalation surrender to the perfect posture and experience it fully.

Work quietly and calmly with direction and certainty.

Observe the breath and keep it smooth and even.

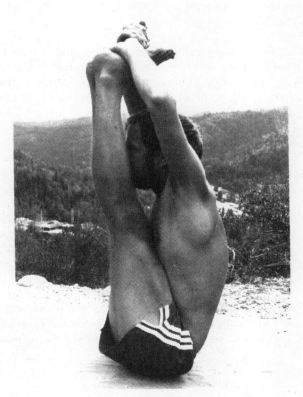

URDHVA MUKHA

PRANAYAM --- HEALTH THROUGH BREATH

The physical postures could be looked at as a reflection of what we express. Pranayama gives an indication as to how we express. Of course, what and how can be seen in all things. However, with the body still, the breath reflects the condition of the mind which describes an action. The mind is the link between initiation and action, and the right or wrong motivation of an action can be seen in the way one breathes. If the breath is jerky, there is a fear or some other disease in the consciousness; and the motivation is therefore not from the true Self that sees with pure vision.

The more deeply we breathe, the more energy we take in. This energy can be an advantage or disadvantage depending upon how we use it. If it is allowed to strain the lungs, draw in negative thoughts or go into useless pursuits, then problems arise. Breathe within the natural capacity of the lungs and increase the energy level in accordance with the ability to be attentive in the breathing practices.

When doing your breathing exercises, it is good to be in front of an open window. The best time to do them is after asanas in the early morning and/or in the evening. Before starting the breathing exercises, it is good to acknowledge the presence of the ONE that allows us to receive the breath of life.

Learn to breathe smoothly and evenly in a relaxed way.

Note the effects of the different types of breathing and use them wherever appropriate. Practice them in the following order:

1) CLEANSING BREATHS (often called fire breathing) quicken the blood flow and eliminate impurities and tensions and they also raise the vibration rate in the consciousness. They increase the active side of brain and body and this can be seen by an increase in dynamism.

2) ENERGIZING BREATHS use Kumbhaka (breath retention) and this helps to vitalize one and develop an inner strength. The effects are seen as a prolonged stillness of the eyes.

3) BALANCING BREATHS use alternate nostril breathing which balances the Shiva/Shakti sides of one's nature. They also balance the emotional and nervous energies. The balance can be checked by an even penetration through both eyes giving even-mindedness and stability.

4) NORMAL BREATHING steadies the body, mind and soul and is seen by a balanced character and personality.

CAUTION: Nature knows where its needs are and balances according to divine laws. Knowledge of these laws, and the application of them, is God's perogative. This is the motivating force in the consciousness of a true Guru and a good teacher. Misuse of certain breathing exercises such as over-holding the breath, or too many repetitions of the fire breath can cause damage, and an imbalance of the energies in the consciousness.

Practice normal breathing and research into the secret of the breath as much as you wish. However, check with a good teacher or make sure that you have contact with the Eternal Teacher within yourself when engaging in any extensive growth practices.

APPLICATION TO LIFE

See if you can work through the levels, using them as stepping stones for the conscious movement of life energy. In making decisions or going with the flow of things:

1) Experience the now (RED)

2) Imagine the perfect state (VIOLET)

3) Observe with inner stillness (INDIGO)

4) Listen to what life is saying (BLUE)

5) Sense the direction in which to go (GREEN)

6) Look at the most suitable steps to take (YELLOW)

7) Concentrate on an aim, letting go of all distractions (ORANGE)

8) Go with the rhythm of life (watch the breath) and enjoy all that you do NOW.

SECTION 3

This section aims at increasing the spiritual values and psychic abilities in the light of new awareness. The subtle forces of nature and their effect upon our state of consciousness are studied at a deeper level. Physical development is approached in a more precise manner, by looking for the basic essential requirements for each posture to encourage the essence (spirit) to flow more easily. The steps of meditation are also introduced as a practical situation to encourage a balanced and a mature spiritual development.

In essence we study: The essentials of Life
The nature of the Soul
Meditation techniques

REFERENCES:
Much of the material in this particular section comes from two sources. For deeper study the following may be obtained from the publishers:

A Course in Direct Perception - 'Into Meditation Now',
by Christopher Hills, 1973.
'Nuclear Evolution: Discovery of the Rainbow Body'
by Christopher Hills, new edition, 1977.

PART 9

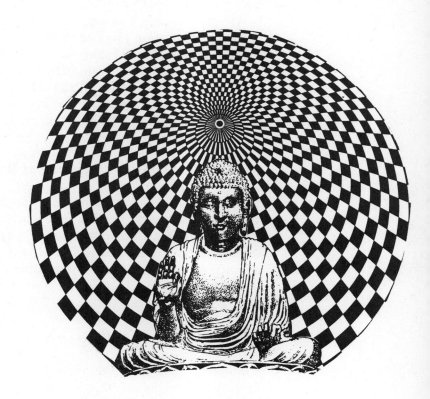

WHOLISTIC
MEDITATION

MEDITATION

Meditation is an action which brings about a realization of the true nature of things and a greater awareness of the SELF who is observing and experiencing what is seen. The meditative state of consciousness is therefore very necessary for effective practical living.

At the beginning of each part of this section there will be a meditation practice that, stage by stage, helps toward establishing a continuous meditative state of consciousness and Self-realization. It is important to realize that truth is always with us here and now and that although there are stages of meditation, truth may be perceived and Self-realization attained at any time since it is beyond time.

Standard Procedure for the Practice of Meditation

When practicing meditation, sit upright, either on a chair or in a suitable posture in which the body can be relaxed around a firm framework of a straight, vertical spine and the collarbone and pelvic rim parallel to the ground. Ensure that the lungs are free from all restrictions in movement. Therefore, keep the knees below the waist.

STAGES OF MEDITATION

Stages 1, 2 and 3 have already been covered in the first two sections of this course. However, a brief summary of them is given below. Study this brief summary and then practice the meditation for this part of the course which uses visualization and is given at the end of the Stage 3 summary:

Stage 1
Aim and Positioning

It is important to know what one is aiming for in life and not to make meditation something separate from everyday living. Ask yourself deeply and often, "What is important? Why am I living?" Discipline your life accordingly.

To be able to hold oneself steady in one's aim, and to maintain a balanced rhythm of incoming and outgoing energy in a chosen situation is the aim of Hatha Yoga. It also provides the necessary foundation for meditation. A regular routine of body postures that will enable you to sit still, stand firm and be flexible in nature is of certain benefit.

Stage 2
Calming and Focusing

After positioning comes a cleansing and quietening process. The breathing exercises of Pranayam (life-energy control) develop this ability. Practice some breathing exercises daily. Watch the breath, listen to it and guide it.

In breathing and in life, focus the attention on the given situation and examine calmly:

What is happening.
How it is happening.
Why it is happening.
Who is making it happen.

Stage 3
Observing and Looking

The practice at this stage is to observe life and one's inner self without reacting or judging and to look with an inner vision at what is being experienced.

Focus the consciousness one-pointedly on a Yantra (a square or centralizing symbol),

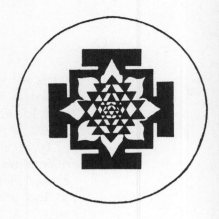

and then on a Mandala (a circle or symbol which encourages the consciousness to expand outward in all directions,

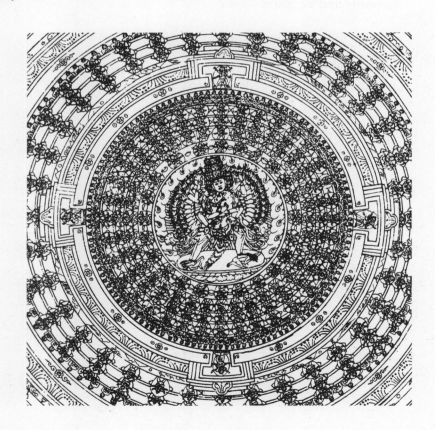

Meditation for Stage 3
Visualization

a) At the point between the eyebrows, visualize the sun in the sky as a symbol of reality. Look how it symbolizes the unconditional radiance of pure consciousness through the vastness of space and imagine the experience of it.

b) Another visualization is on the stature of an enlightened figure. Imagine how such a person's state of consciousness might be.

c) Visualize a stream of water flowing from the hillside through the countryside and eventually into the ocean. Imagine all your desires as being the water of the stream of life flowing into the ocean of love. Feel yourself as a wave of that almighty power of love rising and returning into the ocean depths of stillness.

IMAGINE - MEDITATE - EXPERIENCE - REALIZE!

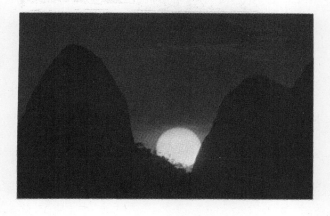

STUDY MATERIAL

THE ESSENTIALS OF LIFE

In section 1 we looked at consciousness in the vertical sense on the physical plane and studied the functions of the seven main areas of the body with their associated glands and organs.

In section 2 we went a stage further and looked at consciousness in the horizontal sense, on the mental/psychological plane. In that section we studied the seven main needs of consciousness with their drives from which the nature of matter is determined.

Here in section 3 we now look at consciousness in a third dimensional sense: on the spiritual plane. This means to study in depth the seven main areas of consciousness at the soul level to find the motivating causations that shape the mind and mold the body.

Diagram 9.1.

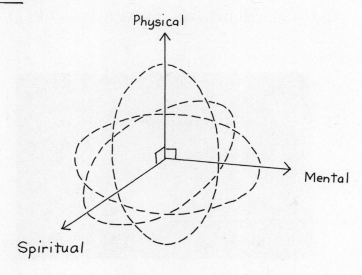

The seven psychological and spiritual centers that we are considering can be located at specific points along the spine of the human body. It must be realized, however, that the mind and soul have no real physical location and are more like fields of energy in communication with as much of the universe as consciousness cares to make them. Only by a concentration of energy and a fixing of it consciously, is matter formed out of spirit. Thus the sensations of time, space and position are given the chance to be identified by the mind. This is the process that takes place through the levels of consciousness from the creating of an imagination to the establishing of it on the physical plane. By relaxing we can reverse the process and experience the finer, expanded fields of vibrating soul energy.

This whole process can be looked at as a circle of life energy flowing in the level of consciousness as shown in diagram 9.2. However, it must be realized that there is a very important vertical component which creates the ascending and descending aspects of consciousness. Together with the cyclic expansion on the horizontal plane, this vertical component helps to form spirals of evolution and involution that create the changes of vibrational level in consciousness.

By keeping the spine vertical and making conscious movements with reference to it, as in yoga postures or spiritual dance movements* (i.e. movements that are made in a balanced state of consciousness), these changes in vibration can be experienced.

In the earth elemental vibration there is a steady feeling. With water, movements are fluid. The quality of fire is dynamic and with the air element, the consciousness is uplifted. In spirit one sees the nature of

*See Rumph Roomph Yoga tape series available from University of the Trees Press.

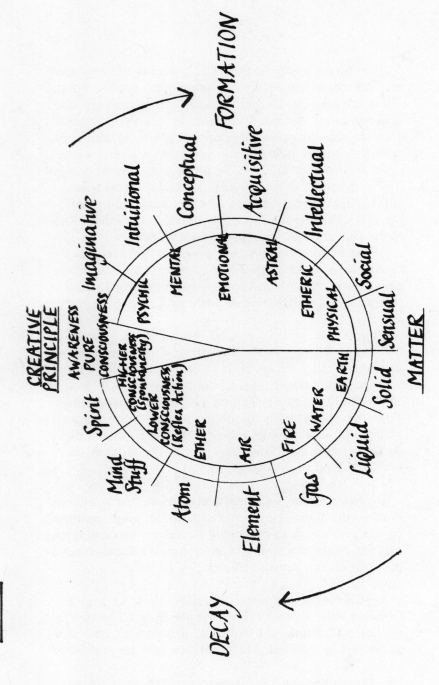

Diagram 9.2.

178

things and in the absolute state there is a union between the state of no-thing and every-thing.

These levels are experienced in deep meditation and through certain exercises which follow later in the course.

The interplay of the triune of natural forces (active, passive and controlling/neutral) expanding and contracting the universal pure energy depicted in diagram 9.2 produces a coil-like formation of energy flow. At the points of intersection of this energy-flow are the chakras (vortexes of revolving energy) which act as vibrating centers of energy for the manifestation of specific actions in life. These points of intersection are centers that can be located in the spine by stimulating the flow of energy in the spine and sensitively becoming aware of the points of intersection that are shown in diagram 9.3.

Diagram 9.3 also shows the formation of chakra points along the spine from the intersection of spiraling life energy. The polarizing effect maintains energy in them and holds them apart, in the same way that circular magnets slotted on a wooden rod are kept apart when the same polarities are facing.

There are many ways of sensing the chakras and studying the effects from them. With a friend you may like to feel the effects in the hands when they are passed over the front and back of the body. Some people can feel cool and warm sensations in the hands over specific points along the body.

If you simply put consciousness into the body at various points along the spine you may become aware of the centers of thought, feeling, imagining, etc. Tense and relax each point indicated in diagram 9.3 and detect any action and reaction in the consciousness.

Diagram 9.3.

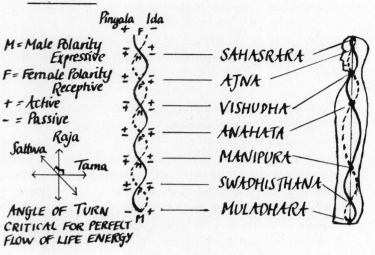

M = Male Polarity Expressive
F = Female Polarity Receptive
+ = Active
− = Passive

Raja
Sattwa
Tama

ANGLE OF TURN
CRITICAL FOR PERFECT
FLOW OF LIFE ENERGY

Pingala   Ida

SAHASRARA
AJNA
VISHUDHA
ANAHATA
MANIPURA
SWADHISTHANA
MULADHARA

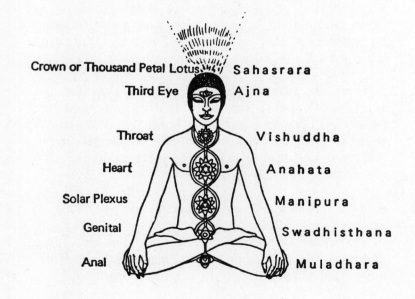

Crown or Thousand Petal Lotus — Sahasrara
Third Eye — Ajna
Throat — Vishuddha
Heart — Anahata
Solar Plexus — Manipura
Genital — Swadhisthana
Anal — Muladhara

Watch carefully the length of the breath as you place the body in the various asanas. Notice the shortness of the breath in the Plough compared with the standing postures. Where the breath goes the consciousness goes and vice versa. See this effect in yourself. Also, in life, look where the consciousness is and how you are breathing. It is by seeing an effect that we can look to the cause and by looking at the nature of the effect, we can discover the nature of the source behind each cause and effect.

Look at the effect of the consciousness when in the presence of a room filled with different colored light. See if any part of the body vibrates with the light. See what is the state of consciousness in the presence of each colored light.

By consciously breathing and directing the attention into the spinal column become aware of the flow of subtle life energy up and down the spine. Along the left psychic channel of the spine (Ida) flows the passive female sensitive current of energy. Along the right psychic channel of the spine (Pingala) flows the active male expressive current of energy. Along the central psychic channel of the spine (Sushumna) is the neutral balancing current of energy. Look into a mirror and see if one eye predominates more than another. If it does it indicates excess of energy flow at that side.

When the currents of energy along the ida and pingala are in balance and the body energy is evenly distributed around the spine, then the consciousness becomes still and union with the creative nuclear self is found. The eyes then penetrate evenly, and the balancing current flows freely and can be directed from the base of the spine up to the crown chakra to produce the blissful state of consciousness called Samadhi.

In each type of energy produced by the chakras there are varying degrees of expanding expression and deepening experience. In the table following are some of these degrees. As you will see, each degree is the effect of another.

Note that in any of these areas or "spaces of consciousness" the energy can be used beneficially or it can be misused to cause deterioration and delusion in the experience of life.

Observe causes and effects with reference to the true purpose of life, to each aspect of it and to the situation that one is in. Look to an ever increasing conscious involvement which faces the situation realistically and brings the love of the One to a higher level. The ability to do this is the art of living and the purpose of Yoga.

When we look to the cause and motivations of our expression, then the degree of awareness increases. What at first may seem just a physical sensation may turn out to be a reflection of a more subtle primal energy that is trying to express itself and fulfill a particular purpose at the moment. If one identifies with the physical sensation alone, that is where the consciousness will stay. To experience a fuller picture of life one needs to understand what is causing these identifications. Look at the whole and see how the consciousness can be directed into the most meaningful realities of life in each particular situation.

If one has experienced a very outgoing life, where the vehicles of sensation have been strongly emphasized, then a more introspective life and contact with the inner self through the vehicle of the "inner" senses would create a more natural balance to life. An introvert may explore the objects of sensation and express himself more fully through the different modes of expression. By reaching out into the physical world, the manifested

INCREASING VIBRATORY RATE

SUSHUMNA

EXPRESSION			PINGALA		IDA		EXPERIENCE	
EFFECT OF SENSATION	VEHICLE FOR SENSING	FUNCTIONAL SYSTEM USED	DRIVE	ASSOCIATED COLOR	URGE	INNER PROCESS	INNER FACULTY	CONSCIOUSNESS
Shape	Brain	Parasympathetic Nervous System	To Create	Violet	To Visualize	Imagination	Realization	Bliss
Form	Eyes	Sympathetic Nervous System	To Look	Indigo	To Idealize	Intuition	Perception	Wisdom
Motion	Nose	Respiration	To Smell	Blue	To Authorize	Conceptual-ization	Recognition	Peace
Action	Ears	Circulation	To Listen	Green	To Secure	Acquisitive-ness	Sensitivity	Love
Speech	Mouth	Digestion	To Taste	Yellow	To Analyze	Intellectual-ization	Discrimination	Awareness
Contact	Skin	Elimination	To Touch	Orange	To Share	Socialization	Expansion	Joy
Regeneration	Sex Organs	Reproduction	To Procreate	Red	To Materialize	Sensation	Unification	Oneness

PHYSICAL REALITY

SPIRITUAL TRUTH

DECREASING VIBRATORY RATE

self can be experienced in a time dimension. By penetrating into the depths of consciousness a timeless dimension can be seen unmanifested. Between the two lies the mystery of life.

In the center of the table above is the pure state of consciousness which reveals that mystery. When seeing with pure vision, experience is no-experience and has no need for qualification or segmentation. However, it is the natural order of consciousness to describe itself by projecting a picture of itself onto the screen of life and then retracing or dissolving that beam of projected consciousness back to itself in the center of stillness. This can be done instantaneously and spontaneously or it can be a gradual formation in terms of time and space. It can also be both.

These dimensions to consciousness lend interest and color to the diversification of the unified state of pure existence. Each level of consciousness has a function in this diversifying process. As long as we can see this functioning and not be identified with it or attached to it, then we can be in conscious contact with the source. It is the ego that separates on the intellectual level and the mind that fixes on the authority level that deludes man in this matter. The heart that wants to possess and the imagination that wants to charm draws consciousness away from the true reality. The lure to the company of society, the excitement of sensation and the falsity of idolizing knowledge for its own sake are all tricks used by consciousness to establish and maintain a creation in time.

If one can see this happening and maintain a pure conscious observation without rejecting the experiences of life, then one can be totally fulfilled in the ONE, without separation, without identification, yet with an experience of life that is ever changing and confirming the Truth of that eternal ONENESS.

Each part of consciousness reflects all aspects in it. The body is a microcosm of the macrocosmic universe and it displays the mind, soul and pure being in its shape, form and material texture. The validity of this statement can be realized through direct perception and through direct experience when the ability to relax consciousness fully and a concentrated effort to evolve beyond the body, ego, mind and senses assists the penetration into the true meaning of things.*

The tracing back of events to the motivations behind actions and thoughts enables one to see ever new reflections of the SELF, this is a love that each individual can contribute to the experience of life and through which others will come to know the SELF.

To know our self more fully by self effort, study and introspection is to love God. To live life more fully by providing the opportunity for others to learn for themselves is the creative way to live and leads to wisdom.

When wisdom and love are centered in the ONE all things are revealed and Peace confirms the presence of the ONE.

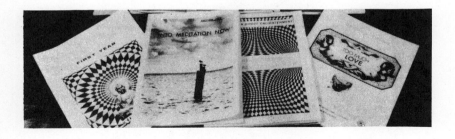

* There is a three-year correspondence course in Direct Perception available from the University of the Trees, to those serious students who are involved in self-discovery.

DAILY PRACTICE FOR PART 9

THEME: OBSERVE WITH LOVE,
LISTEN WITH CARE
EXPRESS FROM THE ESSENCE
THE DIVINITY THAT IS THERE

This part of the course is very much concerned with looking to the essence and using pure imagination to express the absolute. Total relaxation and steady concentration are invaluable to the art of observing and seeing. By observing we can become sensitive to the subtler levels of reality; by seeing we can project into the conscious experience of life a new image of reality.

Pure imagination is the start of the creative process. Create a symbol of an absolute such as wisdom, joy or peace, either by drawing it on a piece of paper or by visualizing it in the mind's eye. Make the symbol simple and draw it from a Center of Being that is absolute. Watch you don't use memory of past events or association with known images. Create it without thought --- use imagination! Use thought and action only to describe it. See if you can use this same process in other ways.

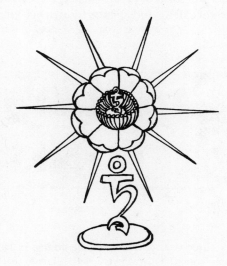

186

POSTURE PRACTICE

In each posture there is an essential feature that is absolutely necessary for the posture to be what it is. An example is Tadasana, the upright standing or mountain pose; in this posture, the ability to stand upright comes from its base, the feet. Without the feet correctly placed on the ground in the right state of "aliveness" the rest of the body will not reflect the essence and meaning of the pose. One could do without the arms and still stand upright. Even a pair of legs without the rest of the body could stand upright on the basis of the feet. This whole posture rests in essence upon the soles of the feet. The positioning of the feet is, therefore, very important. With the body facing forward and the feet together notice what happens when the right foot is turned outwards. See how the body pulls to the right and the whole of the spine is tensed on one side. Even a slight out-of-alignment of the feet or knees with the direction of the body can affect the body adversely. If the body leans forward it can be seen by the movement of the weight onto the toes. Likewise, movement towards the toes affects the straightness of the body. By distributing the weight evenly under the expanded soles of the feet the body becomes balanced. Press equally on the center of the heels and balls of the feet and lift up the center of the ankles: the foundation of the posture is then firm. Spread the skin on the metatarsals and ankles in the natural direction and relax the toes. The posture then has flexibility and character. Practice this pose with the above information. See how you can apply it and then move on to Trikonasana, the triangle pose, and see what you find to be the essential features of that posture before reading the explanation below.

THE ESSENTIALS OF TRIKONASANA

Look at the name of the posture for a clue to its essence. The main triangle of this pose is formed by the legs. Without the legs the triangular base could not be formed to give its very essential feature, which is a firm foundation on which to build the rest of the body and character. The most stable triangle is an equilateral triangle.

Do the pose with the legs only a half meter apart and then 1½ meters apart and notice how different the pose feels. Look where the weight is concentrated in each case. Now place the legs the same distance apart as the length of each leg: an equilateral triangle is formed. Notice this firm base on which to develop the pose.

Make sure that the legs are firm but not rigid and each knee, which is the heart of the leg, is in the same direction as the foot which leads it. Look to the apex of the triangle, the pelvic area, for the motivation in the posture and develop this area for a good communication link between the legs and the body. For a test of balance and to ensure an equal pressure under both feet throughout the posture, practice the posture on a plank of wood balanced in the middle on a wooden block and keep the plank straight throughout the posture. In the following parts of this section the essence of each set of postures will be studied. In the meantime, inquire within yourself what is the essence and the essential feature of the postures and exercises that you do.

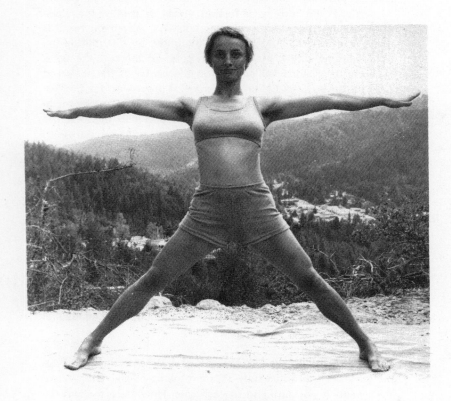

UTTHITA TRIKONASANA

PRANAYAM --- HEALTH THROUGH BREATH
ALL LEVEL BREATHING

VERTICAL BALANCE

1) Sit upright in a relaxed manner. With a metronome or other suitable steady audible beat choose a reasonable count in which you can (a) inhale, (b) hold the breath, (c) exhale, and (d) hold out the breath for an equal count, e.g. 6.6.6.6, 8.8.8.8.

2) Inhale and lift up the center of the front of the body letting the shoulders fall away from the neck.

   Feel the skin and rib cage lifting.

   Think of your highest aspirations and physical well-being.

   Imagine that state of consciousness.

   Reach beyond that state to the state of pure being.

3) Hold in the bliss of fulfillment in the now.

4) Exhale and with the front of the armpits still rising direct the flow of energy down the back.

   Feel all resistance to the upliftment of the body and tensions in the skin relaxing.

   Think of all negativity as falling away.

   Imagine your higher aspirations being brought into manifestation.

   Look to the stillness and peace from the completion of the cycle.

5) Hold out in the contentment of being in the presence of the unmoving undisturbed ONE.

6) Complete 12 of these breaths, maintaining an inner calmness and movement of the lungs without any strain. If the chosen count is too high then reduce it and stay at the reduced rate until the system is truly ready to increase the count. Be wise in your choosing.

Following is an example of how to build up the breathing over a period of days, perhaps weeks --- don't rush it.

EXAMPLE OF A STEP BY STEP SYSTEMATIC APPROACH
(VINYASSA) TO SAMYAMA

Equal Inhalation, (Puraka): Retention (Antar Kumbhaka); Exhalation (Rechaka) and Hold (Bahyi Kumbhaka).

DAY	BREATH COUNT							
	1	2	3	4	5	6-10	11	12
1	8.2.8.2	8.4.8.2	8.4.8.2	8.4.8.4	8.4.8.4	......	8.4.8.2	8.4.8.2
2	8.4.8.2	8.4.8.2	8.4.8.4	8.6.8.4	8.6.8.6	......	8.6.8.4	8.4.8.4
3	8.4.8.4	8.6.8.4	8.6.8.4	8.6.8.6	8.6.8.6	......	8.6.8.4	8.6.8.4
4	8.6.8.4	8.6.8.6	8.6.8.6	8.8.8.6	8.8.8.8	......	8.8.8.6	8.6.8.6
5	8.6.8.6	8.8.8.6	8.8.8.6	8.8.8.8	8.8.8.8	......	8.8.8.8	8.8.8.6
6	8.8.8.6	8.8.8.8.	8.8.8.8.	8.8.8.8	8.8.8.8	......	8.8.8.8	8.8.8.8
7	8.8.8.8	......	......	......	......	......	......	8.8.8.8

The above exercise can be practiced in lying or sitting position.

APPLICATION TO LIFE

The essence of any position in life comes from the essential requirements of the situation. The essence is in the heart of the situation, the center around which other things evolve and cannot be without. Look to the guidance from life by recognizing what the heart of life is expressing through each situation and what it is that has to be learned from it. In a family situation, what is the universal family pattern: What is required of a father, mother, son, daughter, or other role? Also, what is the essence in you that can add a spark of life to the situation? In doing a job or anything else in life, look to the essence of it for the realization of Truth and Love.

PART 10

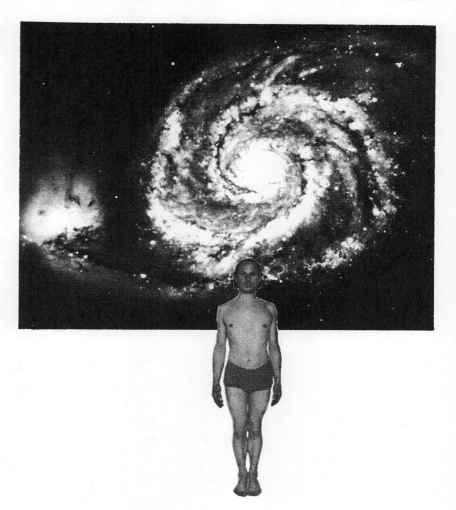

CREATION OF THE WHOLE BEING

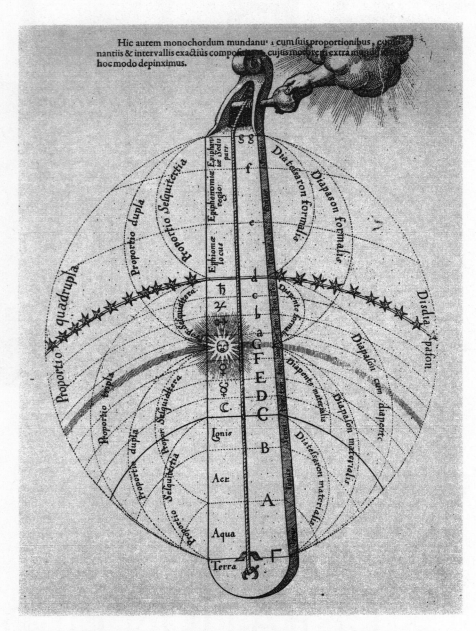

GOD'S HAND tunes the "monochord of the world" in an illustration from a book published in 1617. The classical elements and the planets appear, along with the musical ratios.

MEDITATION PRACTICE
CHANTING AND MANTRA

This is the fourth stage in the understanding and development of consciousness through meditation and it deals with listening and hearing. By totally absorbing oneself in a sound, it is possible to go beyond the sound and any thought of hearing it. Consciousness is being put into every sound we hear and it is consciousness that is listening to every sound that we make. All states of consciousness come originally from a pure state. In chanting and listening to a Mantra we listen for the pure sound in all sounds and learn to recognize the same essence behind all sounds. Put another way, we use the mind to transcend the mind by keeping it focused on the eternal and hence protecting the mind from straying into delusion (MAN - TRA : mind - protection).

CHANTING

Chanting consists of repeating words or a sound with deep attention until one reaches the essence of the sound and meaning behind the words. In chanting, the repetitions are vocalized by in-toning in the throat until the tone produces harmonics, called sruttis, which resonate with the tone and can be heard as high-pitched sounds, yet they are outside the normal range of the human voice. The most well-known chant is of the word AUM, which means the ALL IN ONE. That is, the creating of vibration, the maintaining of it and the dissolving of it back into the silence, is of the ONE SOURCE.

MEDITATIONS

1) Chant freely and with attention the word AUM or ONG. As you chant, let the word fall out of your mouth and listen from the source of the sound. You may start with a groan and gradually build it up to a positive tone. Vary the shaping of the throat

and lips until there is a good round and refined sound, unwavering and expanding in all directions. Go with the sound, listening all the time for those high-pitched sruttis and the constant deep whirring motor-like sound which keeps energy in the sound.

2) A slight extension of the last chant is the Tibetan Chant AUM MANI PADME HUM, pronounced OM MANI PEDMI HUM, and means "the all-in-one is the jewel in the heart of the lotus and is my True Self." In other words, the priceless, all-pervading essence that brings out the beauty of the white lotus flower from the muddy waters in which it grows is similarly unfolding in me.

At the end of a chant, spend some time in silence listening for the "ringing" sound within.

3) One can also chant with any sound one hears from the whirring of an engine to the sound of a note on an instrument to the spontaneous sounds of the environment.

MANTRA

Mantra is silent chanting and is done mentally. Eventually one lets go of the sound or just loses it as the consciousness is absorbed in the essence of the sound within.

Some sounds like RA and MA encourage the manifestation of a universal consciousness. RAMA is the God (vibration) of action and this mantra can help one to work more effectively. It can help to "earth" one.

SA lifts the consciousness and HA creates a warm and joyful expression.

EE as in "peace" broadens the consciousness in a horizontal sense and increases tolerance.

194

MEDITATIONS

1) Find your own mantra by becoming very still and listening within to what your essence is saying. What is most meaningful to you? Do you hear a direct vibration, a singing sound, a word or a phrase?

2) Repeat a sound or words that draw you to your center.

3) Listen to the sounds of words that describe the absolute to you. Perhaps the sound of words like love, wisdom, peace or joy ring a note of truth in you.

Repeat chants and mantras for long periods of time until you really go into the essence of the sound.

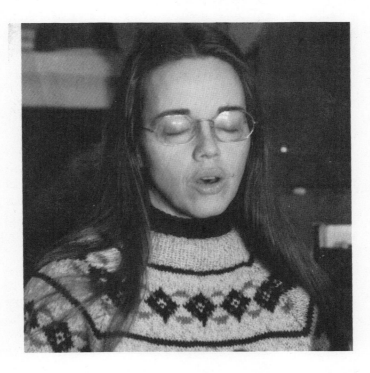

STUDY MATERIAL

THE BEGINNING OF EVOLUTION

The whole of creation and its evolution is linked by consciousness and is contained in every part of it, just as in every leaf of a tree the Source of life is moving the life energy through the sap and creating the many unique patterns of energy in the leaf itself.

Through this love of the universe in which each part is given the intelligence and energy nourishment to create itself, yet be ever guided by the Source to a state of fulfillment, man is able to contact his creator within his own consciousness and become "at-one" with the creator of all. When man has learned to make this contact by meditation he can come to know the mysteries of the universe and experience the all-pervading, all-knowing, all-powerful, ever loving, ever blissful state of consciousness which, in Sanskrit, is called Satchittananda - Truth, pure mind, blissful love. This attunement can be attained through action and by looking at life and living it from the perspective of the all-encompassing ONE. By uplifting the deluded soul so that the physical manifestation is in true harmony with the ONE, Yoga is realized.

In meditation (meaning wisdom - action) one learns how to see the Truth and how to manifest this perfect state through Yoga at the same time. Since the perfect and the imperfect (order and chaos) are reflected in all parts of creation we can learn to see the nature of the creator by understanding the creation.

To understand creation fully we need to go back to the beginning of creation within ourself and see how the Spirit of consciousness filters the images of perfection and imperfection down into a physical reality and also what conscious energy drives the physical reality back to the reality of a pure state of existence that is still, at peace, and beyond the consciousness of creation. What is it that interferes with this natural process? Let us now examine the process of natural evolution.

1) Relax deeply into a state of stillness. Relax the body until there is no association with it. Relax the mind until there is no thought and the mind has the freedom to detach itself from any limiting conditions. Relax the soul until there is no identification, association or condition left in the consciousness; the consciousness is pure and eternal; existence is a stillness that is at peace with itself.

2) When you have reached this state, let the idea of movement filter into the consciousness and then return to the stillness again.

3) Now become aware of the breath with a movement which expands and a movement which contracts, without reference to anything but its own projection of thought and its return back to the state of nothing. This is a vibration and a wave of energy.

4) Begin to be conscious of the breath in the nostrils and the sensation of coolness with the inhalation and warmth with the exhalation.

5) Now center yourself in the throat and listen to the SA-HA sound of the breath in the throat as you close it slightly. Notice how you can observe the vibration and how you can use it as a projection from yourself.

6) Experience the movement of the lungs and feel the body breathing. With the movement, notice how association takes place.

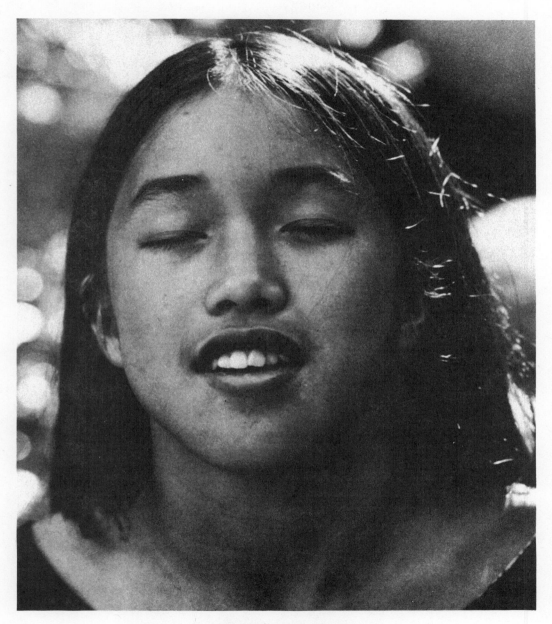

AM I WHO I THINK I AM?

7) Take the breath into every part of the body and stretch it in the inhalation and relax again on the exhalation. Notice how the consciousness locates itself in form and shape and establishes the physical reality relating to it and recreating it in physical and social order.

Now go back into breathing consciously in the lungs and notice how life in the body is dependent upon this action.

Then put the consciousness into the throat and notice as you listen to the sound how the control of that sound controls the way the lungs expand and contract and hence affects the body. Close the throat and notice how the throat has the authority to determine life in the lower parts of the body and the state of them.

Next put the attention in the nostrils and notice how the direction of the breath up the nostrils affects the sound of it. Aim the consciousness into the bridge of the nose and direct the breath into the head. Notice not only the lightness but also notice the disassociation with the rest of the body. Block up the nose and see how this area has control over the throat and lower parts of the body.

Aim the consciousness above the head and see how you can lose consciousness of the body and go into a trance state beyond the body. This process can be continued until the consciousness enters a state of blissful stillness, yet vibrating in a finely attuned, balanced state of oneness or wholeness. Any distraction from this balance separates the consciousness and the relationship of I and That produces duality and relativity. Study your own consciousness to see how this state comes about and what it is that colors the consciousness. Become aware of the formation of the ego and its pure purpose. Go beyond the balanced blissful state to the void beyond vibration and see the Self return in the stillness of the relaxed state, but on another level of awareness.

The stages of the development of consciousness through the mind, ego, body and senses are told in the story of Genesis and its return is told in Revelations. In between are the scriptures that describe its many-faceted nature and the guidelines for its evolution. As conciousness begins to vibrate from a still state, each movement of consciousness creates a dimension of time and space. Hence we have the days of creation as periods of time, yet they can be realized and experienced in everyday life, every hour, every minute and every second, since creation, maintenance and dissolution is a cyclic process that comes with every experience which relates to a time space world.

Let us now look at these stages or days with reference to the psychological states already discussed and with reference to the build-up of the reflection of an image, projected onto a screen with the aid of a light source and a light-converging lens. See page following.

You will notice in the relaxation earlier and in watching the breath, that there is a natural cycle of events in the life process. In this cycle, the all-pervading life energy can be focused and built up with an individualized nature, form and shape. Also, this energy can be maintained and dissolved back into the ground state of pure energy, like waves of the sea. Each breath, each wave of energy is different, yet all movement takes on a common cause of events. The effect is an ever-changing experience of life which can be stored, reproduced and forgotten by the consciousness that created it. However, the final pattern of creating, projecting creation onto the screen of life and returning to the ground state, remains an eternal pattern which continues as long as there is conscious energy, awareness and will power to fulfill it.

DAY	ANALOGY WITH PROJECTOR	STATE OF CONSCIOUSNESS		STAGES OF CREATION
		Ascending → Individual Soul	Descending → Universal Soul	
0.	(Source)	I am.	Pure Consciousness.	Void – no movement.
1.	Picture of Self. Self Seeing	<u>Desire to Replicate self.</u>	<u>Image of Perfection</u> Oneness and pure state of I AM which embraces all. ABSOLUTE	<u>FORMATION OF LIGHT</u> Projection of I AM image (Word of God).
2.	Self Forming Image	<u>Desire to Share</u>	Idea of earth, water, fire, air and ether principle. IDEATIONAL	<u>FORMATION OF DUALITY</u> Observation – detachment from idea (void). Will – Idea of creation (projection of image I
3.	Image Projecting	<u>Desire to Change</u> replication and creation.	Conceptualising the elements of creation. MENTAL	<u>FORMATION OF MINERALS & VEGETATION</u> Feeling of ALL IS ME.
4.		<u>Desire to Acquire</u> or to own total universe.	Securing or establishing, through vital force, the elements of creation. EMOTIONAL	<u>FORMATION OF HARMONY</u> Sensitivity / Experience Receptive / Expressive

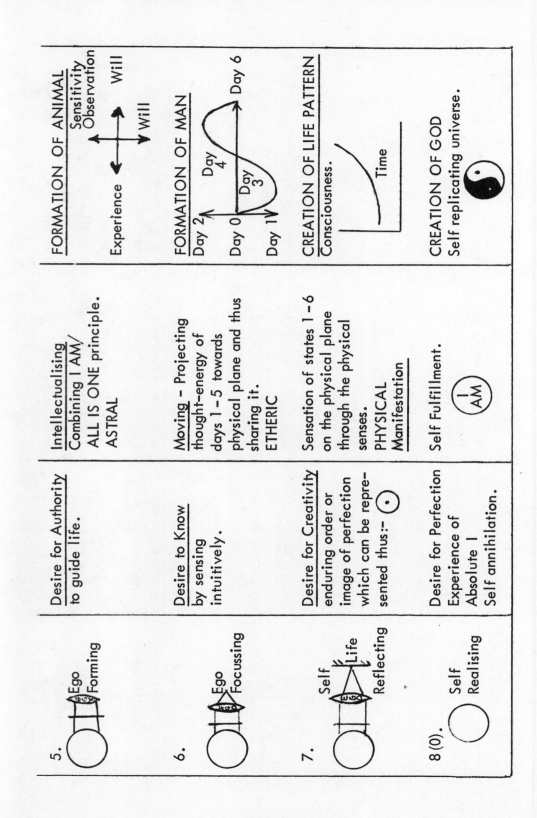

5. Ego Forming

Desire for Authority to guide life.

Intellectualising
Combining I AM/ ALL IS ONE principle. ASTRAL

FORMATION OF ANIMAL
Sensitivity
Observation
Experience
Will / Will

6. Ego Focussing

Desire to Know by sensing intuitively.

Moving – Projecting thought-energy of days 1–5 towards physical plane and thus sharing it. ETHERIC

FORMATION OF MAN
Day 2 — Day 0 — Day 1 — Day 3 — Day 4 — Day 6

7. Self Life Reflecting

Desire for Creativity enduring order or image of perfection which can be represented thus:– ⊙

Sensation of states 1–6 on the physical plane through the physical senses. PHYSICAL Manifestation

CREATION OF LIFE PATTERN
Consciousness.
Time

8 (0). Self Realising

Desire for Perfection Experience of Absolute I Self annihilation.

Self Fulfillment. (I AM)

CREATION OF GOD
Self replicating universe.

It is by surrender to the ONE who is beyond creation and by upliftment to the state of pure undifferentiated consciousness that one can learn how to follow the natural patterns of creativity and use the primal energies in an evolutionary way. Consciousness is then brought to a higher level and degree of manifestation. The more pure consciousness that is put into anything, the more effect it has on the whole. In other words the more selfless, conscious involvement there is in anything the more beneficial the eventual outcome. Remove the blocks of self-limitation and pure consciousness flows freely.

On a universal scale consciousness is evolving in cycles of time on all levels, physical, mental and spiritual. In the human body too, cells are evolving in cycles of time on all levels. On each level patterns of energy repeat themselves until their readiness to increase vibration and come to a more subtle level of consciousness is reached.

Change comes about through the breathing process, by the universe expanding and contracting, or an individual's movement of the lungs. In the human body see how the lungs expand and contract with the breath and how performance of the body is affected by it. Breath entering the lungs through the throat can be controlled by the throat positioning and can affect the movement of the lungs. The way the breath enters the nostrils will affect the way it enters the throat and so forth. On the mind level, thoughts can affect the breath and vice versa. Note how states of joy, fear, calmness and excitation affect it.

The pranayam exercises of yoga are ways of increasing the evolution process of the body cells and hence the consciousness will be able to see the effects of this. By observing consciousness in actions and reactions in moods, and in the mind's delusive nature, the enlightened state begins to unfold. Remember, however, that the physical environment and the universe around us is not evolving at the same rate. This seeming wide gap between heightened awareness and the seeming lack of change in the world around may cause intolerance, confusion or other reaction which, again, brings delusion if it is not understood and approached from a centered viewpoint. Therefore, always meditate on the Center. Be still within and see all with a pure consciousness — unreactive, undisturbed and untainted by judgements or conditions, assumptions or projections. Be centered in the oneness and learn by looking and practicing, hearing, and speaking Truth with a sensitive awareness to the nature of things.

Perhaps one of the most obvious experiences of vibration is that of sound. In the human voice are many vibrations and in toning one can hear sounds outside of the normal human voice range. These very high and low vibrations are revealed in toning by tuning to the heart of the sound one is making. Toning in unison with a sound encourages a union with the heart of the sound when one listens intently. Vibrating the note deeper and deeper in the throat refines the sound and takes the consciousness into its essence.

Each note has its own vibration characteristic. Go into this by listening carefully with a sensitive inner ear to the harmonics in the note and the effects that the note has on experience.

Every vibration has a definable and indefinable quality. Every posture has its definable shape yet every person will put their own individuality into it. A posture done with full consciousness into the whole of it will show more life than a posture that is done with only shape as the motivation. Every situation in life requires one to hold a certain attitude. The one who is centered will be aware of that attitude in his being. The beatitude of the consciousness experiencing the situation is shown by the fruit of the action. A person who is centered will bring forth love and wisdom in every situation. The uninitiated will bring forth chaos and dissolution. Three notes on a musical instrument can be played mechanically and they will not move anyone to dance or change their consciousness. The same notes can be played musically and life energy will radiate through the ear and uplift those who have ears to distinguish the vibration as a spontaneous outflow from the source. Indeed, the whole of life is alive here and now with the sound of music. If one can transcend the delusive nature, the mechanical and the musical will be seen playing hand in hand, in time to the baton of the ONE who conducts the whole ensemble of vibrations.

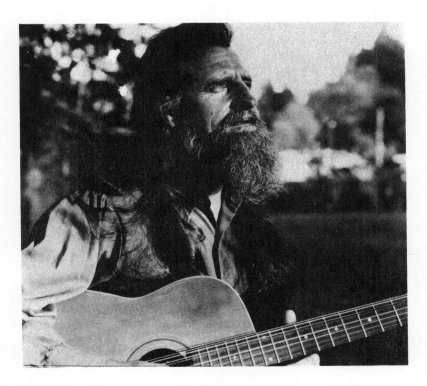

CHRISTOPHER HILLS: CHANTING FROM THE HEART CENTER

DAILY PRACTICE FOR PART 10

THEME: FEEL WITHOUT DESIRE,
THE SOUL'S CEASELESS YEARNING.
BE OPEN TO THE TRUTH,
WITH ATTENTION ON TRUE LEARNING.

Listening to the Truth by being still within and looking from an objective point of view at the consequences of an action can reveal the real desires of the soul.

On the surface it may feel comfortable or even right to continue a certain habit. A feeling of not wanting to bother about doing a certain job of work can easily be rationalized by the mind into the excuse of "going with the flow" of the heart. If this happens a few times, look at the pattern developing in consciousness. Is not wanting to bother the real feeling? Look at the effect of continuing this pattern and the effect of changing that passive state into an active willingness to work with a caring attitude.

This exercise of extending with the imagination the consequences of an action to its ultimate conclusion can help to develop both effective patterns of living and of posture. Learn to change any negative resistance into a positive assistance to the soul's true motivation. Focus into the real direction of the heart and face it intelligently with the head.

POSTURE PRACTICE --- INVERTED POSTURES

In the last part of this section we began to look for the essence in the various types of posture by seeing what are the essential features that bring out the true nature of each posture. In other words what parts of the body make the posture what it is and how do these parts need to be positioned in order to provide a good foundation for the positioning of the rest of the body? In the standing postures, you will remember that the essential features are the feet and legs. By focusing the attention into the correct positioning of these parts and lifting up the front of the body, the essence of the posture is brought out from the Muladhara chakra.

Now we look at the essential features of inverted postures and what it is that brings out the essence in these positions.

206

SARVANGASANA --- NECK BALANCE

Although this posture is normally called the shoulderstand, the title Neck Balance is more appropriate, since the essential feature is the balance of the body on the neck and the lift up the back of the body from the neck.

For the energy to be focused into the neck and throat and for the essence to emerge effectively from the Vishuddha chakra up the body into the legs and toes, the positioning of the head, neck and shoulders is very important.

Before going up into the posture make sure that the shoulders are pulled well away from the head and the elbows pulled well away from the shoulders. Turn the palms to face upwards with the little fingers higher than the thumbs so that the elbows are brought close in to the body and the shoulders brought flat on to the ground. Take the energy into the spine between the neck and shoulderblades.

On the exhalation, raise the legs, making sure that the head is extended fully away from the body and is completely relaxed. The effect of the body weight and the inner relaxation together tone the Thyroid and Parathyroid glands. When this meditative state of consciousness is directed up the body and the body is held in a balanced position, levity equals the challenge of gravity, and an inner strength develops in the consciousness. The essence of the posture can then be realized and experienced.

For lasting effects maintain the balance for some time. For perfect balance it is important that the elbows are kept well in, such that the center of the upper arms and elbows rests on the ground. This helps to bring the consciousess into the shoulder-blades and up the spine. If weight is felt on the inner edges of the upper arms, the energy will tend to move out to the shoulders and push the elbows outwards, resulting in the posture collapsing. When there is perfect balance the elbows and arms have no weight on them and they act merely as a guide for the positioning of the trunk.

Lifting the energy from the neck and shoulders and directing it up the spine, the sides of the body and into the straightening of the legs, encourages the divine qualities of wisdom and compassion.

207

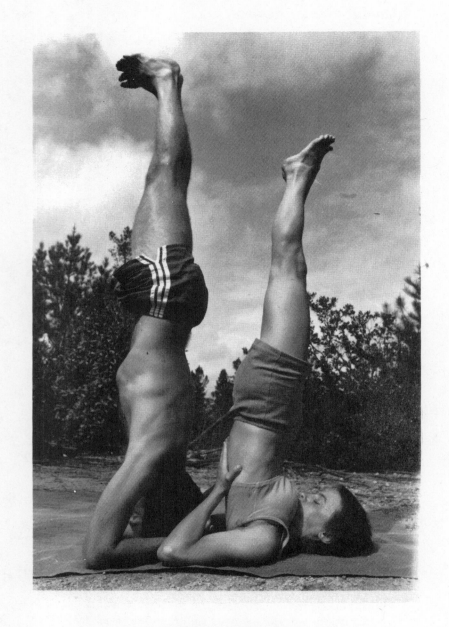

SIRSASANA and SARVANGASANA

SIRSHASANA - HEADSTAND

As with the neck balance, the essential features of the posture are the head and neck positions so that the energy is taken up the spine and in toward the center of the body and thereby encouraging the consciousness to turn inwards. Focus the attention into balancing on the crown of the head (Sahasrara Chakra) and keeping the nape of the neck (Ajna Chakra) relaxed but firm. The eyebrows should be parallel to the ground. With the head too much on the back, the neck becomes tight. With the head positioned too much toward the forehead the neck arches and the skin then is too soft. The arching also reflects with a bowing in the lumbar region.

The weight on the forearms and elbows needs to be in the center of them, not on the outer edges. The elbows also need to be in line with the shoulders and the wrists need to be well apart. The hands form a wall against which the back of the head touches only the thumbs. The wrists need to stand vertical to the ground. The shoulders need to be lifted by pressing on the center of the forearms. Bring the dorsal region in and the waist back.

Again, the balance and an upward lift up the spine bring out the essence of the posture which encourages intelligence and the power of objective perception. There is also a regenerative effect on the pineal and pituitary glands.

PRANAYAM: HEALTH THROUGH BREATH
ALL LEVEL BREATHING
HORIZONTAL BALANCE

1)   Sit upright in a relaxed manner.

2)   Inhale and expand the sides of the body from the waist up to the shoulders. Feel the skin spreading to the outer edges of the back and front. Think of all the finer qualities of life such as wisdom and peace permeating the universe. Imagine all thoughts and feelings being used by the universal Principal. Experience the expansiveness of a stage of consciousness that is open.

3)   Hold for a moment in the fullness of the breath.

4) On the exhalation, contract the sides of the body from the shoulders to the waist. Feel the skin going in toward the spine. Think of all the finer qualities of life such as love and joy being absorbed into the body.

5) Hold out for a moment in the perfection of stillness.

6) Complete 12 of these breaths.

APPLICATION TO LIFE

The mechanical element of life is guided by the universal intelligence of logic and reason.

The spontaneous element flows from the freedom to explore and from the love of change. Together in perfect union, ever new harmony and creativity shine forth. Separated from their true union, law is necessary and chaos is ever lurking in the shadows of ignorance. In consciousness there are aspects of the higher, lighter Self and of the lower limiting self. The conscious ONE sees all aspects at play and guides them according to the situation at hand so that the union of the positive elements is expressed in love, awareness and creativity. The negative aspects are disciplined and returned to the source of stillness in order to emerge in a new light. Positive and negative are ever changing as the nature of the ONE is expressed in polarity (diversity) and experienced in unity (purity).

Look at every situation from the center of consciousness and uplift it in an evolutionary way so that life can revolve on a new level.

PART 11

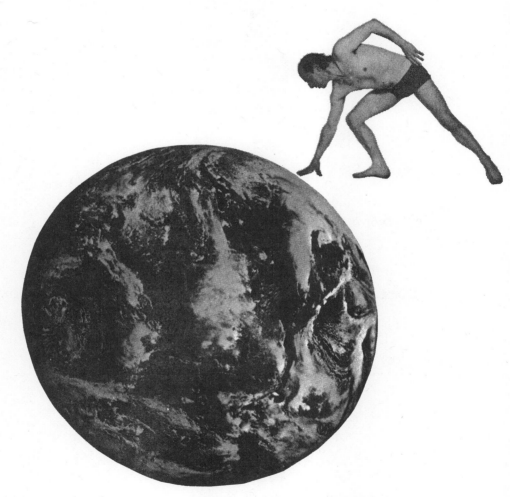

HEALTH AND THE
BREATH OF LIFE

MEDITATION PRACTICE - ATTUNEMENT

The fifth stage of meditation is attunement and affirmation. Attunement is a state of resonance and balance between receptivity and expression to such a degree that there is a unity between the creative principal and the patterns of nature. Man is a pattern of nature and when there is a balance of the energy, awareness and will power in man, then his center of consciousness is also the center of consciousness for his higher Self, the universal creative force. This is shown in the diagram below which includes the directives that help to bring it about.

Diagram 11.1.

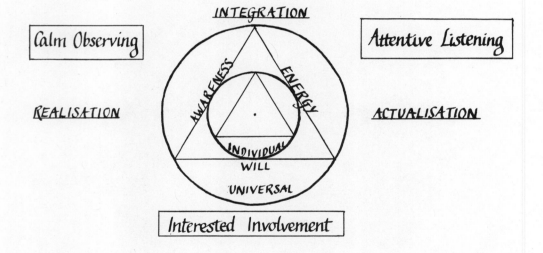

When awareness, energy and self-will are balanced, the triangle is equilateral and the center of individual consciousness (inscribed circle) is the same as that of the universal consciousness.

In life, attunement comes when anything is done with an involved interest backed by a calm enthusiasm, an awareness of the needs surrounding the situation, and a careful attention that brings out the best from the situation unconditionally.

Practice the following meditation using the sounds suggested and then expand it into a meditation on the sound of life as it presents itself to you.

At any moment, tune in to the vibration of the situation and to the people concerned with it.

MEDITATION

Attune to Truth by visualizing and observing, chanting and listening at the same time, until the consciousness is completely absorbed in the object of visualization or the essence of the chanted sound. When the consciousness is tending to go inwards to the centered self, a vibration of HUM or ONG can assist it. When the consciousness is expanding, the vibration of AA or OO helps it to be so.

Attunement is a refining process, a perfecting of a situation or condition with consideration for the whole.

Some of the subjective effects of attunement are:

An increase in energy level.
A feeling of expansiveness.
An inner peace.
An awareness of the fine detail and subtler vibrations of consciousness.
A recognition of the presence of a unifying force in life.

When you find a state of attunement, hold on to the experience with an affirmation of the Truth.

ALL IS WELL; ALL WORKS FOR GOOD.

STUDY MATERIAL

THE CYCLE OF LIFE

In meditation the consciousness can be calmed to a void of stillness or it can be vibrated to a balanced state of heightened awareness.

In the calming process a state of consciousness can be reached in which there is almost a sleep state. The point at which there is just sufficient awareness to hear the sounds around one, and yet see the pictures of the subconscious mind, is called the state of Yoga Nidra.

Diagram 11.2.

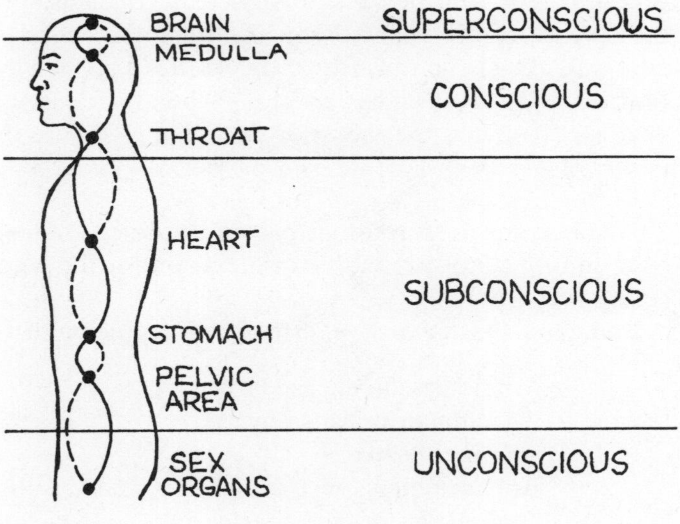

This realm of the subconscious can sometimes be seen when one is just beginning to wake out of sleep and is aware of dreaming. Look at these dreams, they show the workings of the subconscious mind which play back the contents of the conscious mind, together with images, situations and associations from past events. The passive state of Yoga Nidra is normally a relaxed state. However, by letting the mind become drowsy and then breathing slightly through the nostrils with a cool breath, the observer of consciousness is awakened enough to experience the thoughts and images of the subconscious mind.

To see the unconscious mind, look into the reactions in the mind when there is a stress situation or pain in the consciousness. Notice what comes to the surface of the consciousness. By facing what is normally difficult to face, the unconscious mind emerges with the causation of those difficulties and the seeing of this may lead one to the discrimination between false identification with the ego and the true nature of the SELF.

A very open, spaced-out type of relaxed meditation can also bring out the images of the unconscious in imaginary fantasies and nightmarish pictures. If these effects become a problem, focus the consciousness into something practical: some service to others, or some worthwhile project in which enthusiasm and interest can assist the focusing on Truth. The use of throat breathing (SA - HA sound) can also help to "ground" oneself.

The conscious mind can be seen directly by looking at how the consciousness experiences the now. See what is important to you by seeing what you are doing now. How is it being done? See the motive behind it.

To see the superconscious mind, deep concentration and the ability to project oneself out of the confines of body consciousness is necessary. Pure imagination and intense listening can provide an openness without expectation and a sensitivity that is receptive to new experiences which come with superconsciousness.

Life flows in cycles; aspiring up to become super-conscious, thoughts and energies are drawn up from the subconscious mind. Replaced in the subconscious mind are memories of conscious experiences and glimpses of the superconscious vision. This apparent up and down movement and cycle of energy sends waves of manifested energy out in a horizontal and lateral sense (like a cork sends out waves when it is bobbing up and down in water) and these reflect the superconscious, conscious, and unconscious mind as experiences of life, while the subconscious mind absorbs and stores the information for replay at a later date, often as dreams during sleep.

If you look at a coin you will find that you can only look at one side directly at a time. The coin of life is likewise: we may look consciously with our eyes and mind and directly perceive what is before us. To see the other side of life directly, however, we have to turn our consciousness inwards and face the other side of ourself directly.

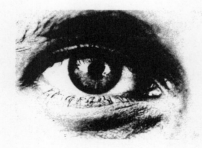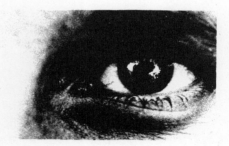

Now, though we can see only one side of a coin directly, we can know to some extent what it is like on the other side at the same time as we look at the side facing us, by:

Using the memory of similar coins that we have experienced in the past.

Feeling with the fingers to obtain an impression of the other side.

Using a mirror to reflect the contents of the back. Note, however, that the mirror gives a laterally inversed image.

By looking at ourself, our actions, thoughts and ways of doing things, we can look back down the beam of consciousness and obtain an impression and feeling of what we are really like.

By looking at life around us and seeing our reactions to how others do things, and to what life is presenting to us, we can see a reflection of our other side.

In a posture, by using our eyes and hands, we can see and feel shape and form. By feeling at the back or by doing a posture, we can detect if one part of the body is more or less tense than the other, and gauge when both are balanced and correctly aligned.

By using a mirror we can see the shape at the back and, also, with two mirrors, we can see the front and back.

By looking for the essential features of a posture and aligning the body according to them, the Truth of a united individual with a universal order can be seen. In Trikonasana, when the legs form an equilateral triangle, and the spine is made parallel to the ground, the straightened spine forms a tangent at right angles to the inscribed circle of the equilateral triangle. (See diagram 11.3.)

Diagram 11.3.

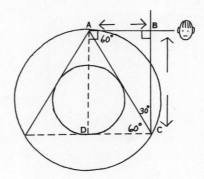

The symmetry of such a pose reflects the Truth of order and proportion in the universe. The right angles of the body shape on the physical vibratory sphere resonate with the mental vibration associated with the right angle of view for a straight ordered mind. Such a mind resonates with the archetypal image of the triangle in the soul and sees the equality of the right that all things have to existence. The rectangle "ABCD" lifts the soul's earth quality, establishing a stable even-mindedness and a right use of the physical energies.

Balance of the body around its center line and a correct proportioning of body parts along the center line bring harmony into the body and "uplift" it. Centering the consciousness and putting it into every aspect of a situation, the direction that will most uplift that situation will be revealed.

A calm observing of the flow of life through the body brings an understanding of its ways and its nature. A calm observing of the life around one brings an understanding of the reason for living, and reflects the nature of oneself. The development of a true society begins with this understanding of oneself.

Experiment with each area of the body. By directing the breath into the coccygeal, sacral, lumber, dorsal, cervical, medulla and brow areas, the chakras can be "tuned up". You may notice, as you direct the breath in this manner, how it twists and spirals up and down the spine in the way of the Caduseus shown earlier in this section. The angle at which the column of energy enters and leaves each chakra center is very important to the tuning of it. Like water flowing into a plughole, the spiral shape increases with the correct flow, control and conditions. The tuning process is a very subtle operation, and a tremendous awareness, plus the balance of concentration to relaxation is necessary.

The best way to start tuning the chakras by breath control is to balance the breath as it enters through the nostrils and through the throat as described in the earlier part of the course. Nostril breathing increases awareness in the consciousness. Throat breathing increases the control of the will to take energy into the body. Careful lung movement determines the quality of the energy. The balance of the cool and warm sensation of the breath at the top of the nostrils and inside the head balances the Ajna and Sahasrara chakras. The balance of the cool and warm sensations in the throat and heart balances the Vishuddha and Anahata chakras. Breathing with a deep, equal expansion and contraction of the lungs brings a union and balance between energy and awareness. By ensuring that the will does not force the breath or allow the attention to lapse, balance of the will with energy and awareness brings about attunement of the individual and universal Self.

Continuing this process further into the abdomen, pelvic and anal regions, the Manipura, Swadisthana and Muladhara energies are brought into attunement. The superconscious, conscious, subconscious and unconscious selves thereby find peace. The wholeness of the individual and the universe can then be realized. What is seen in the body is seen as a principle of the workings of the Universe and of each cell of the body.

Another way of tuning is by toning a note AA or ONG and directing the consciousness inwards to the center of the note. At the same time listen to the wholeness of the sound and encourage a fullness in it.

Again, by putting the attention in different areas of the body, the chakras can be located by different notes and, in each area, there is a note that resonates exactly with that area. Toning during posture work can help to release inner tensions and be a guide as to when the consciousness is calm and attuned. If a warbling sound or excessive variations in pitch of the sound are experienced, a strain and out-of-attunement with the true SELF is indicated. Toning a pure, whole sound when in a posture can bring extra life into the body.

Looking inwards, listen to the silence in the center of the sound within. Listen expansively and aim for the note that brings out the most harmonics --- the high pitched, silky sounds (sruttis). Also, feel the low energizing vibrations. Merge with the whole sound.

I AM THE LIGHT OF THE WORLD

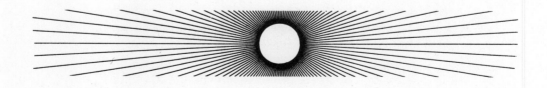

DAILY PRACTICE FOR PART 11

THEME:
SIT WITH THE SOUL IN THE CENTER OF LIFE
AND MEDITATE ON THE MEANING OF SOUND
AND OF LIGHT

In life there is always a way of seeing things from another perspective. By recognizing what is not true in a situation one can work in other directions until the one that shows truth reveals itself. By looking to the way of the masters, and by having a reference within oneself, such as an inner calm or state of being at ease, then any off-centeredness will immediately throw up into the mind signals showing a need for change. Without that change there will be a sense of dis-ease and, indeed, disease will result if conflict remains in the consciousness. Situations that bear the fruits of growth with ease can bring encouragement and confidence into the mind, and to others. This courage and confidence can also be a foundation for tackling more difficult situations which, before, may have created limitations and lethargy.

When difficult situations become easy, growth is taking place.

When problems are seen to contain their own solution, intelligence is increasing.

When all situations, problems, and limitations are seen as being self-made and changeable, then the mysteries of life unfold.

POSTURE PRACTICE --- Twists

The essential feature of all twisting postures is the spiralling action of the spine, starting at the sacrum and continuing up the spine. This makes the nervous system more flexible, expanding the inner consciousness and increasing the sensitivity to contact in more parts of the body. Mental activity is stimulated and a more acute attitude of mind is encouraged.

The essential body parts of all twists is the spine and, in particular, the sacrum and buttocks. Keep the two buttock bones pressed equally on the ground and, with the sacrum pointing upwards, make this triangle of three points the basis on which to lift the spine perpendicular to the ground. With the waist slightly forward, extend up the spine, focusing the energy into the sacrum (Swadhisthana Chakra), the middle of the lumbar (Manipura Chakra) and the middle of the dorsal (Anahata Chakra). The essence of the posture flows from these points upwards and outwards into the arms and into action as the spine and body are lifted and turned. The external effect is to thin the waist and broaden across the front of the shoulders.

The twisting postures encourage a raising of standards and the development of fine detail in thought and actions.

SITTING FORWARD BENDS

The essential features of the sitting foward bending postures are the parts which sit on the ground --- the back of the legs --- and the parts which bend --- the pelvic basin and the sacrum area. When energy is focused into these areas (Mulhadara and Swadisthana Chakras), the essence of the posture can emerge. The spine is made to elongate and come parallel to the ground. The head is dropped in a passive state. The results are a quietening of physical and sexual activity, a calming of emotions, and a relaxation of the mind energies.

PASCHIMOTTANASANA

Noting what has been said above, make sure that the back of the legs are flat on the ground, especially behind the knees. Extend the heels and the inner edges of the legs so that the sacrum and waist are brought forward. See that the soles of the feet are flat with the toes pointing directly upright. Notice how this brings energy and life into the base of the spine and sacrum.

Lift the spine upright, take the pubis back, and bring the waist forward. Lift the tailbone so that the sacrum comes down. Extend up the front of the body on each inhalation. Straighten the spine and surrender the head to the toes on the exhalation. Drop the head and work quietly in the posture by repeating the above directions until no more extension is possible without strain. Then relax more and more deeply in the posture while maintaining the extended position of the body.

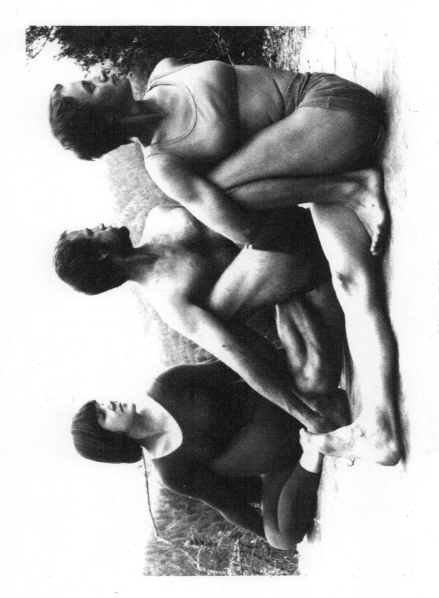

SPINAL TWIST

PRANAYAM - HEALTH THROUGH BREATH

1) Sit upright with a straight spine and collarbone horizontal to the ground. Become used to the firm cross-like structure of the spine and collarbone (+). Let the skin of the body form around it in a relaxed way.

2) Breath as for normal breathing and then be conscious of the following expansions and contractions.

SHIVA BREATH

3) On the inhalation expand the consciousness and imagine yourself becoming the whole universe of pure life energy. Hold only for a moment.

4) Drop the head as in Jalabandha and on the exhalation let all the energy of the universe come into the body and to all parts of your being, uplifting them to their fullest stature.

SHAKTI BREATH

5) Keep the head dropped as in Jalabandha and on the inhalation let your consciousness penetrate to the center of the still, pure life energy within as the breath enters the body and your being. Hold only for a moment.

6) Lift the head to face forward and on the exhalation, surrender that pure life energy to the wholeness of the universe with a sense of serving the ONE source that provides and protects all things.

7) Repeat (1) and (7) ten times.

8) Relax and breathe normally.

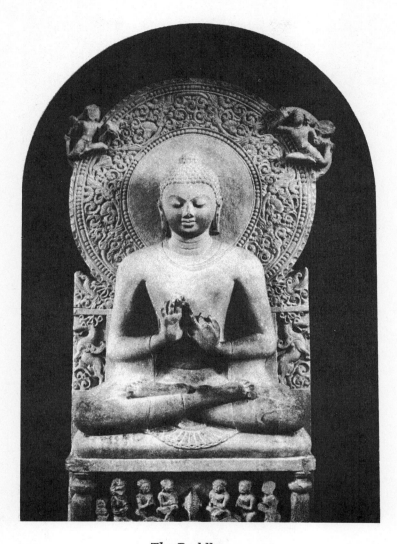

The Buddha

In Buddhism the concept of a personal God does not exist because all entities are created and experienced in our consciousness. The Buddha is a symbol for the pure unconditioned consciousness beyond thought where only awareness of eternal oneness exists.

APPLICATION TO LIFE

The heart is the motivator of life energy and stimulates the expression (sound) of the one who is living.

The head is the vehicle for the light of awareness of the one who is seeing life.

Together with direction from the one with a purpose, life evolves to an ever greater fulfillment and vision.

With the head and the heart in true marriage, in accord with the true purpose of life, pure consciousness is ever present.

Flowing spontaneously with an intelligent approach to each situation in life will provide a direction and balance in all that one does. Balancing the active and passive elements of our nature with due control and flow is the science and art of yoga. When true purpose is behind an action and it is done meaningfully, a positive outcome is seen and felt. This feeling and recognition is the experience of the word (vibration) of God. Bringing the refinements of precision and perception into daily work with joy in the soul is living consciously in attunement with the word and with God. You may not realize when you are in this attuned state. However, if you have been in it, you will know when you are out of it. Having tasted "It", nothing else outside of "It" will satisfy the soul.

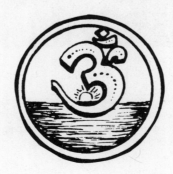

PART 12

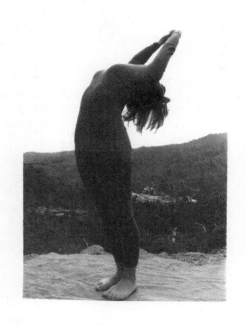

WHOLISTIC LIVING AND DIRECT PERCEPTION

MEDITATION PRACTICE
EXPANDING AWARENESS

From the effects of attunement practiced in part 10 we come to the sixth stage of meditation which is "Realization and Direction". This means the realization that the Self is not separate from anything of which it is conscious. The self who is attuning consciousness is motivated by the same source (Self) who is being attuned to with consciousness.

If you feel well and say to yourself "I feel well" and then if someone else says to you "You look well", who is the one who is listening to those words? Who is experiencing the cause and effect that the words describe? Is there any difference in the recognition of the feeling when it is expressed in the mind and when it is receiving recognition in the mind by the same words spoken by another person? Who is feeling well and who is seeing you as looking well? Is it not consciousness that is seeing from both sides? Then who is the ONE who is creating the thought in the conscious minds of both parties? Is there one mind?

MEDITATION

Imagine yourself in all things and all things as in your consciousness, not outside of it. Now practice dissolving the one Self into people, plants, suns and planets to the extent that you can feel how another feels, think the way another thinks and do what another person does. Do whatever has to be done from the viewpoint of all things being as one SELF. Look for the true nature of each part within that wholeness.

Direct your life according to the realizations that come to you. The effects of your realizations can have a great influence upon the lives of others. At the same time others may affect and influence you, positively or adversely. When dealing with people or with situations, see what is required for the true essence to emerge.

228

STUDY MATERIAL

SUMMARY OF SECTION 3

Here we come to the "nitty gritty" of meditation. With the process of meditation comes the realization that the whole of nature can be experienced in consciousness. Consciousness of breathing is consciousness of life with its evolving and involving effects which spring from the same source.

Take a blown-up balloon as a representation of consciousness and whatever changes are made to its shape at any one point, such as pulling it up at the top into a sausage shape, or poking a finger into the side of it, the rest of the balloon is affected in some way. To bring it back into shape, whether the changing force has to be removed or a complete reshaping has to be done, every part is again affected.

In meditation, acknowledgement must first be given to the source that creates the consciousness that is aware of itself. The more one goes into the silence and the stillness, the more the unfathomable reveals itself and the more one can experience the presence of the ONE. Realizing the dependence upon an ever-deepening source for existence and life, the meditator grows in humility and is ever open to a Universal Principle that gives meaning to life beyond the cause and effect principle of Karmic Law.

With individual consciousness one has the freedom of observation and the responsibility of unifying experiences which govern actions and reactions. With universal consciousness one has the freedom of experience and the purpose of diversifying consciousness into a new set of values and patterns.

As seen earlier in this section, each part of consciousness has a true purpose that encourages evolution with an energy that manifests positively as creativity and a sense of heightened vibration and lightness. The opposite resistive element to this evolving process is a restricting delusive force which involves energy negatively in a destructive manner to the extent of experiencing a lifeless state of consciousness in ignorance of anything outside of the tensions of the body, confusions of the mind and limitations of a conditioned soul.

Direction in life comes from the source within all things. When this direction is not followed, pain from conflict between direction and manifestation results. The ego forms out of a separating nature that analyzes and discriminates. Wrong discrimination brings pain, right discrimination necessitates a follow-through in time, of that which seeks manifestation. The thinking mind focuses upon and establishes whatever it sees to be valid. When ego and mind are understood they can be used by the higher SELF for evolutionary and revolutionary purposes. When not understood, involution takes place and the ego and mind are involuntarily let loose in consciousness. Once identification with these involuntary actions takes place, delusion takes over.

On every level the separating, delusive force encroaches on the growing process and needs controlling by reference to the center within and the situation around one. For example, in breathing there is a subtle state of control. Just letting the breathing happen can encourage laziness and may allow all sorts of variations to disrupt a smooth, equal inhalation/exhalation. A quick thought can affect the breath and a sudden disruption in the breathing may cause a reaction in the mind. On the other hand, making the breathing happen can encourage aggression or it may create a state of dull mechanical repetition without the spontaneity of change and natural life force expansion. Between these two approaches is a balanced state where all is done from a state of consciousness that experiences no-thing being done since there is no "I" to separate itself from the action and everything that is done. The result of this attunement is an increase in energy when it is needed and a stillness of the energy when it is not needing outward manifestation. To maintain this state means a constant vigil to ensure that the ego does not attach itself to false identifications and so create delusive mind impressions which condition the self and limit expansion and creativity.

An example of this limiting action of a negative ego and the creative delaying action of a positive ego is as follows:

An imaginary person called Jack is hungry. This is a natrual condition and a function of the digestive system is to send the signals of hunger into the conscious mind.

Now say someone calls and needs Jack's help just as he sits down to eat. Although Jack's stomach needs food to fulfill its function of transforming food energy into other forms of energy, timing is important and consideration of the whole is the governing factor in the situation. The positive use of the ego would be to delay the eating process until after the visitor has been seen. The negative use of the ego would be to ignore the cry at the door for the sake of satisfying the body with food there and then. There may be several approaches to this situation.

What is important is the concern for the self which includes the needs of the visitor and also Jack's needs. One may have to be sacrificed for the other or by the delaying of an action. If Jack were absolutely on his death bed for lack of food, then that would be most important, since without life in Jack he cannot help the visitor. However, Jack must truly be honest and sincere with himself before a creative outcome can result. Helping another with resentment is no better than not helping at all. An evolutionary outcome would result from willing more energy and using it willingly to master the situation.

An example of the delusive force playing through the mind is when wants are interpreted as needs. Again the circumstances of the situation at hand give the guideline. In one situation a car may be nice to ride in but it may not be a need. In another situation it may be essential for the transportation of the body in the most effective way.

Another trick of the delusive mind is to imagine one is called upon to provide help or healing. An extreme example is when someone is in pain. To try to remove the pain, give advice, or take the case in hand without truly knowing the cause, is the ego at play.

A guideline here is to ask:

Am I qualified to deal with this need?

Is there anyone else around who can deal with it more effectively?

Isolated with a person in need, one may have to give first aid help. However, if the person needs a more qualified service such as a doctor's ability, a social worker's knowledge or a spiritual teacher's advice, then the egoless way to deal with the situation would be to guide the person to an appropriate counsellor.

The polarities of positive and negative energy, male and female expression, are relative and provide points of view which vary from individual to individual. All may be right from their own viewpoint. What spiritual growth is all about is going beyond the points of view, to the fulfillment of the real need in each situation so that the situation reflects a spontaneous flow of Love or a universal pattern or law. Spirituality means a mastering of the egocentricities, assumption-making processes, mind-limiting associations and false ego-identifications. It may be a painful process, yet it can be a refreshing process, a purification, a tuning-up and a re-directing of life energy onto a new level of love.

Spiritual growth will mean facing fears, doubts and the negative side of oneself. Go through it and there comes forth the inner sureness, confidence and new understanding that knows without trying to know, that does without effort, and that has without having to look for anything.

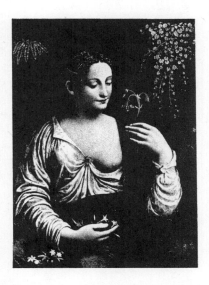

Da Vinci's visual concept of serene
confidence.

SUMMARY OF DAILY PRACTICES FOR PART 12

THEME:
LOSE ATTACHMENTS TO TENSIONS
DON'T IDENTIFY WITH UNLASTING COMFORTS.
LIFT CONSCIOUSNESS TO THE HIGHER
*   INDIFFERENCE*
AND FEEL THE HEART OF THE IMMORTAL
*   ESSENCE.*

It is looking at oneself and life from a heightened perspective that allows us to see things in their proper place. The physical plane is but a small part of total experience and is unlasting in its nature. It is not until the non-attached perspective is attained that experience on the physical plane has true meaning. Identification with the physical plane creates an imbalance with the rest of our being --- hence, dis-ease. True fulfillment on the physical plane comes about when it is seen as a reflection of the spiritual ecstasy from union with the creator. To let go of the ego and attachment to mind and body is the ingoing aspect of growth. To express the true pattern of life through these aspects is the outgoing aspect of growth. The balance of these brings union with the ONE.

POSTURE PRACTICE --- Backbends

The essential features of Backbends are the hollowing of the lumbar region and the extension of the front of the body so as to draw the shoulderblades at the back into the heart and lung region (Anahata and Manipura chakras). It is from here that the essence of the posture emerges to excite the heart and lungs and stimulate the ability to express activity.

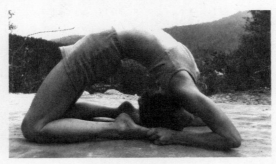

KAPOTASANA

234

CHAKRASANA

In backbends such as Chakrasana where the feet and hands are on the ground, the feet and hands need to be in line with the shoulders and the feet parallel to each other.

By lifting up the front of the legs and pressing the heels on the ground, the sacrum is lifted and the chest and sternum are brought forward over the wrists.

In backbends such as Dhanurasana the lift up the front of the body and the lift-up of the legs gives a less vigorous effect than Chakrasana. Nevertheless, in both the above cases the expressive energy is channeled towards a complete circle from head to heels, a reflection of the "wheel of life".

LYING DOWN POSTURES

In lying down postures such as Savasana (passive) and Jathara Parivartanasana (active) correct positioning of the spine flat on the ground allows a relaxation and rejuvenation of the body, mind and soul. However, it is important to realize that the lying down postures require as much detailed alignment as any other posture and a conscious effort is necessary in order for the essence of the posture to emerge.

SAVASANA

Both sides of the body must lie equally flat on the ground. In Savasana the feet need to fall away from the center line of the body at an equal angle, as also do the knees. See that the buttocks go away from the sacrum towards the heels. See that the shoulder-blades are tucked in and the bottom of the shoulderblades point to the sacrum. Turning the palms upwards, bring the shoulders flat to the ground.

Make sure that the head is in line with the body and the nose in line with the navel. Make sure that the underside of the chin is vertical to the ground so that there is no tension caused by a stretched throat or tucked-in chin. Let the eyebrows move away from each other and let the skin on the brow move away from the center of the brow. Lift the hairline, relax the face and relax the hair on the head.

By relaxing tensions and redistributing the energy into a balanced field of undisturbed vibrations, peace flows.

UPRIGHT SITTING (MEDITATION) POSTURES

Upright sitting postures such as Padmasana and Virasana need practice. The necessary alertness and steadiness for meditation is encouraged by the straight spine and steady base of this kind of posture. The upper legs need to go down and away from the body to give complete freedom to the breathing; a cushion is often a useful asset for these postures. When the body is still and correctly positioned, a still, yet vibrant, state of consciousness is attained.

PADMASANA

The beauty of the lotus pose is seen and experienced in the positioning of the legs, spine and head, such that a perfect isosceles triangle with equal sides and a firm base is formed with the hands placed in Jnana Mudra on the knees.

The feet need to cross the center line of the body without any wrinkles in the heel. The straight spine and upright head allow the subtle psychic nerve currents to flow freely up and down the Ida and Pingala nadis in the spine. This unifies the energy of sensation at the base of the spine with the energy of initiation at the top of the head. When currents and energies are balanced, a heightened sense of awareness is experienced. In this way the consciousness is lifted out of the limitations of body confinement into the realms of immortal Spirit.

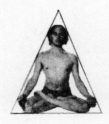

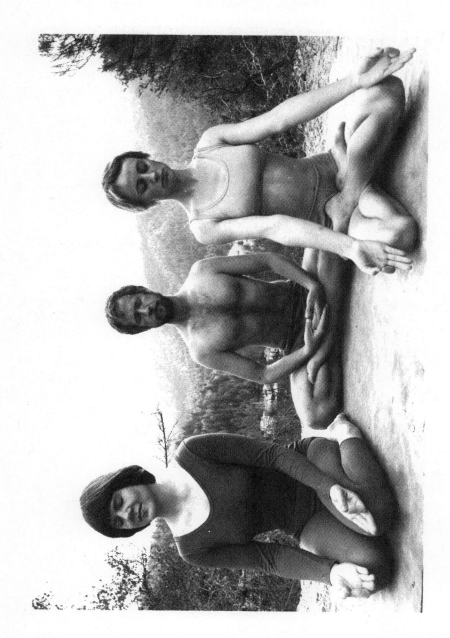

PADMASANA

HALF-LOTUS

VIRASANA

PRANAYAM: HEALTH THROUGH BREATH
ALL LEVEL BALANCED BREATHING

This exercise combines the balancing of energies between the vertical sense (physical), horizontal sense (mental) and spherical sense (spiritual). It also balances the Shiva/ Shakti energies.

1) Sit upright in meditative posture, watch the breath, and breathe smoothly and evenly in tune with the natural rhythm of the breath.

2) Balance and equalize:
   a) the cool sensation in the nostrils on the inhalation with the warm sensation in the nostrils on the exhalation, and
   b) the SA sound in the throat on the inhalation with the HA sound on the exhalation.
   c) the expansion of the lungs on the inhalation with the contraction of the lungs on the exhalation.

Combine a), b) and c) for six full breaths.

3) With the above balance and equalization combine the pranayam exercises of parts 9 and 10 so that:
   a) on the inhalation, energy rises up the center of the front of the body, while the sides of the body expand sideways from the waist to the shoulders, and
   b) on the exhalation, energy moves down the center of the back while the sides of the body contract from the shoulders to the waist.

Observe the flow of life energy from the perfect still center of consciousness. Experience the fullness and expansiveness of Universal love in the breathing. Complete six breaths.

4) On the inhalation expand the consciousness in all directions into the universe. At the same time, surrender to the deep, still center within. On the exhalation bring the energy absorbed from the universe into the body, mind and soul, to uplift them. At the same time, surrender all actions, thought and feelings to the wholeness of the universe. Repeat six times.

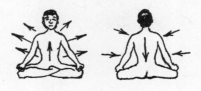

238

SUMMARY OF THE ESSENTIALS
OF DAILY YOGA PRACTICE

YOGA means literally "Uniting with the Source".

To experience the essence of this statement in daily life is to experience the presence of a unifying factor in all things and to realize the diverse expressions of life as a total expression of oneself. The realization of the self as one with the Source of Life is the aim of meditation. The knowing of the self through a conscious movement and balance of life energy is the aim of yoga practice.

LIFE is the experience of conscious vibrating energy, willed into patterns and form with observing awareness.

CONSCIOUSNESS is what we see with and what is seen.

Both yoga and meditation practice involve the study of consciousness and the laws (ways) by which we see with it. In the diagram below consciousness is depicted with its basic parameters geometrically.

Diagram 12.1.

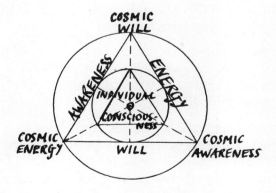

239

What can be seen impersonally on a scientific basis can also be directly related to on a personal level by experience and vice-versa.

In its pure state, consciousness is undefinable. Identified as everything, it is attached to no-thing.

In the deluded state, consciousness identifies with the patterns of energy and form at the expense of awareness.

In yoga the balance of all energies with the awareness of their cause and effect brings about the peace of knowing and the security of absolute freedom from identification. Control is thereby possible.

LAWS OF CONSCIOUSNESS for study and realization in yoga practice and everyday living are:

> Consciousness goes where we put it.
> Consciousness sees only what is of itself.
> Consciousness evolves according to the interest in it and the willingness to grow by it.

THE ESSENCE OF CONSCIOUSNESS is in the observing, listening, still center of the SELF from which all life evolves, revolves and involves itself.

THE KNOWING OF THE SELF comes from finding the joy in moving consciousness.

In the experience of life, discriminate:
> what is permanent, what is passing,
> what is natural, what is habitual,
> what is conditional, what is essential.

See each situation as it really is:
> listen to that which is important in each moment of the now,
> do that which can be done willingly, together with
> doing that which has to be done in the situation for the common good of all.

The essential of daily yoga living is the spontaneous application of knowledge and practice to life as a whole. Whether we develop the body, the mind, the soul or a situation in life, in every position there is a state of consciousness and a way of doing things that brings about the most beneficial effects. If, in the consciousness, there are reactions, then the Ego is speaking. If one is minding what is done, or being done, then the mind has taken over. When one does what has to be done and sees what is being done as a cause for a better understanding of life, then the SELF is expressing freely and direct perception can take place.

DIRECT PERCEPTION is:

when the self sees all things as itself. The consciousness is then pure. When the self moves consciousness to reflect a greater awareness and ability God is then glorified. When awareness and ability are shared with all as oneself, True love is then exemplified.*

DIRECT EXPERIENCE is:

present with the elimination of separation.
When the SELF is known, God is known. When the conscious is still and devoted to the ONE, the presence of God can be felt.

The way to gain direct experience can be shown, but the actual experience cannot be given. Only the opportunity to receive can be shared. Therefore the heart of the devoted yoga student goes to the essence of what the wise ones say and do. He then sees that essence in himself and how life is reflecting it to him through them.

*The University of the Trees offers a correspondence course in direct perception called 'Into Meditation Now'. This is a three-year program for serious students of consciousness only.

SECTION 4

This last section of the course gives a summary of what has gone before and a direction for further unfoldment and discovery. It deals with the minute and infinite, the microcosmic and macrocosmic aspects of consciousness. With any growth comes added responsibility in life and a guideline for the wise channelling of this maturity is suggested. This includes:

The use of Maps of Consciousness
Seeing the Unity of all paths
The right use of Individual choice and
    Universal Guidance

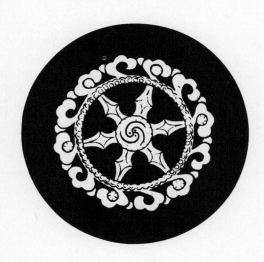

PART 13

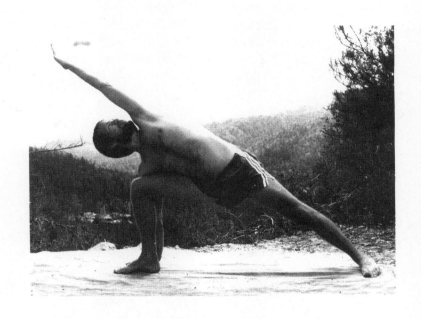

MAPS OF INNER SPACE

MEDITATION PRACTICE
ALL LEVEL MEDITATION

Realization and direction is one thing, actualizing and integrating it into a pattern of living is another. This final stage of meditation (stage 7) emphasizes action in a certain way. This way is to learn how to remain centered at all times while going about doing the work of the day. To tune to the true motive of all actions and to either let things be or to confront the doer with a sensitive awareness of each situation and of each one's relationship to it. If there is any reaction in the consciousness it must be calmed, centered and understood before true communication can take place.

Learn to move consciousness with ease onto all levels by practicing the following meditation:

MEDITATION

Sitting in meditation posture, direct the consciousness to the base of the spine and, while visualizing the color red, look at what motivates your actions. Listen to physical sounds, either in the body or around you, and sense the temperature of the skin on the body. Put your consciousness into the study of the physical level and what it means to you. What and how do you like to express on the physical plane? How important is it in your experience of Truth and Love?

Repeat this study, focusing the consciousness onto each level in turn and at the appropriate place in the body and the spinal column. To remind you of the colors and corresponding parts of the body resonant with the levels of consciousness, a map of consciousness follows (diagram 13.1.)

Diagram 13.1.

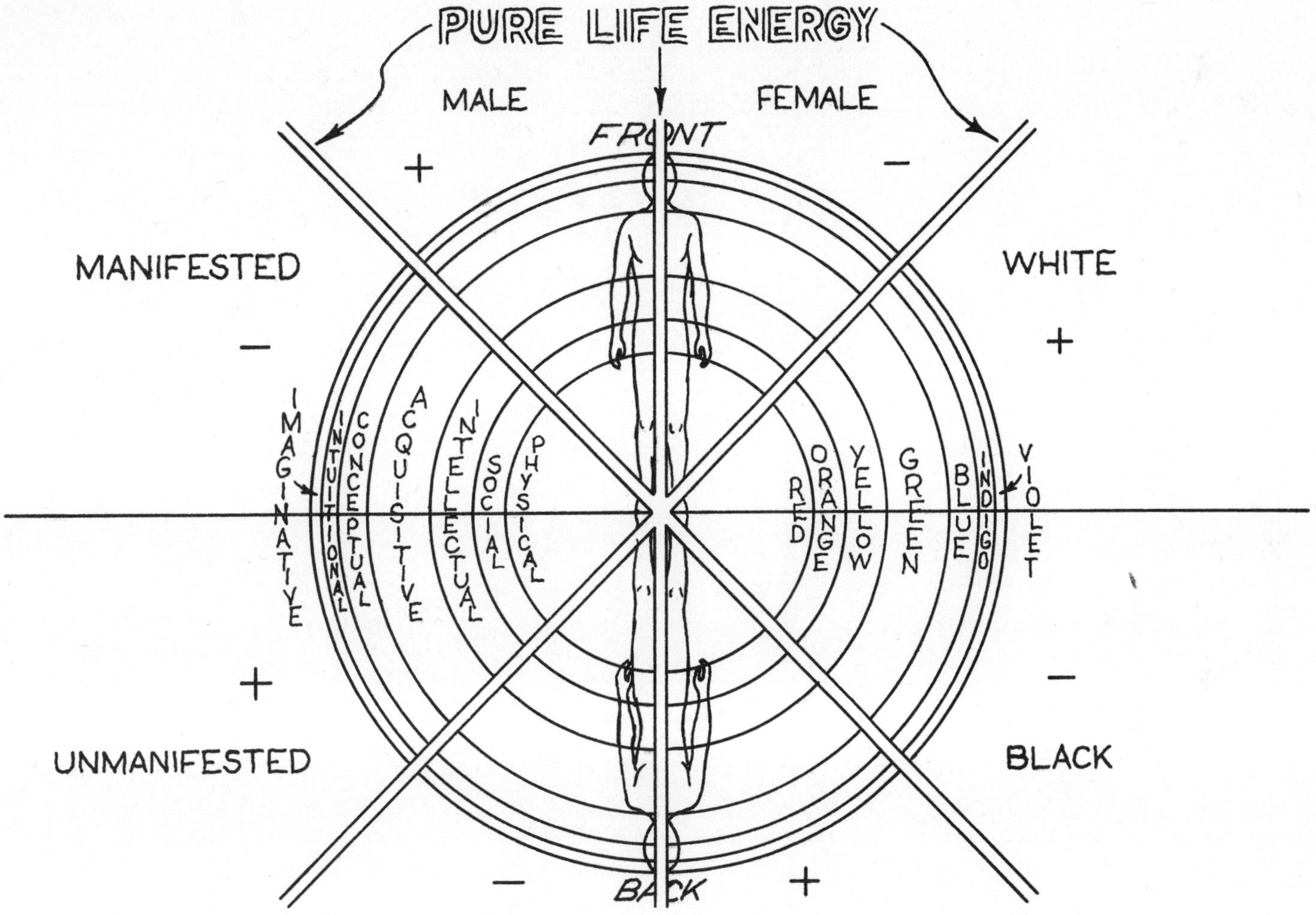

PURE LIFE ENERGY

WHITE +

BLACK −

FEMALE −

MALE +

MANIFESTED −

UNMANIFESTED +

FRONT

BACK

VIOLET
INDIGO
BLUE
GREEN
YELLOW
ORANGE
RED

PHYSICAL
SOCIAL
INTELLECTUAL
ACQUISITIVE
CONCEPTUAL
IMAGINATIVE

THE ELEMENTS OF MEDITATION PRACTICE

The elements Earth, Water, Fire, Air and Ether are types of vibrations which create form in consciousness. Certain postures resonate with the elements and amplify their effect.

Earth Form

The consciousness that is into earthliness is firm and fixed in the direction that it is aimed. Standing postures re-enforce the vibrations of the earth element.

Water Form

The consciousness that is of water nature is flowing and sees the cyclic patterns of energy flow as life's meaning. Forward-bends re-enforce the vibrations of the water element.

Fire Form

The consciousness that is firey is passionate and easily able to rouse energy for the purpose of furthering a cause or expanding a theme. Twisting postures encourage the rousing.

Air Form

The consciousness that is airy is light and musical in expressing the drama of life through movement and upliftment. The shape of backbends brings out this elemental vibration.

Ether Form

The consciousness that is etheric is refined, out-reaching and imaginative in describing the essence of life's message. Inverted postures resonate with this vibration.

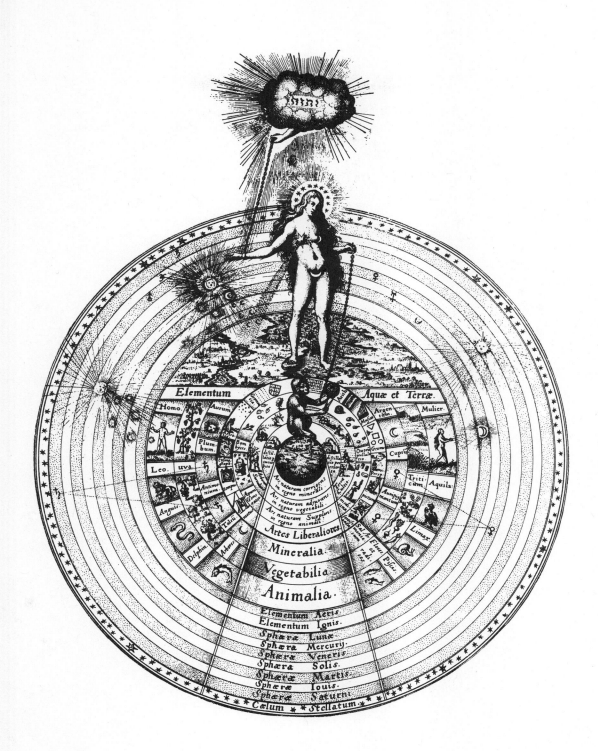

DAILY MEDITATION PRACTICE

In a daily practice of meditation it is an advantage to include all the above elements in the form of a framework for consciousness to both challenge itself and to open itself to the true spirit and nature of the ONE. Combine all the stages of meditation in the elemental framework.

EARTH   Start your meditation exercise with a fixed concentration exercise. Listening to a sound, visualizing a yantra, or the toning of a mantra, are all methods of 'earthing' the consciousness and developing the way to focus consciousness in a fixed direction.

WATER   Next, watch the thoughts that come into the mind. Follow the ideas or feelings to their source and to their fulfillment. See the patterns of consciousness that emerge and the ways of looking at life from many angles.

FIRE   Follow the above practice with the application of fixed concentration to the study of Truth in any area in which you are particularly interested and can easily arouse enthusiasm and willingness to work sincerely. The working through a holy book such as the Bible, the Bhagavad Gita or the study of the 'Into Meditation Now' course are examples of this kind of study.

AIR   Let the Being flow spontaneously. Let the imagination wonder, express in art, science or other areas whatever you would like to communicate to God and to the world. Don't let the lower self make any excuse about not being able to draw, or play an instrument; simply do it in the best way you can. Develop it further, with the spontaneous flow of ideas, images, thoughts, feelings and actions which are centered in the essence of life.

ETHER Attempt the impossible --- experience being a flower, another type of person, being the whole world with people and your own body as cells in a planetary Being. Have the responsibility that God has in seeing all as one. Do not doubt, yet do not be egotistical. Simply Be!, without a self-conscious "I".

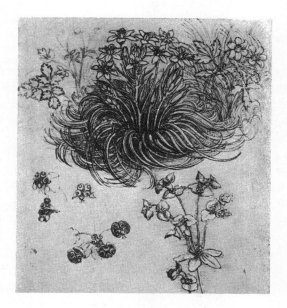

LEONARDO
Star-of-Bethlehem

LIVING MEDITATION

After the practice of the above spend a few moments relaxing and see what is necessary for the day --- what is important? What has to be done? Start your day with direction but be flexible where you can and be open to change without becoming disturbed. Bring anything that goes "out of hand" back into line, which requires the skill of a meditative mind. See if what you would like to do can be incorporated in the day's work. It may be writing, drawing, wood work, or anything that is very interesting to you. Write down the needs of the day and see if you can fulfill them.

STUDY MATERIAL

THE USE OF MAPS OF CONSCIOUSNESS

In the analysis or examination of consciousness we can look at it as a whole, look at it with two sides, or we can cut it into threes, fours, fives, etc. All parts have their relevance in some way or other. The ONE is in all parts and the nature of all parts is in the ONE.

So far, we have emphasized the ONENESS of all things and the POLARITY or twoness within all things. When balancing polarity in the triangle of consciousness through energy, awareness and will, we attune to the TRINITY of the ONE.

With the study of the effects of posture on consciousness we studied the sense of upward, downward and side to side flow of energy. In other words, the FOUR-FOLD nature of consciousness expressing itself.

Looking inwards, the reference of the fourway expression to an inner Center brought a FIVE-FOLD look at consciousness. The five pointed star is a symbol of this. The human body as seen with a head, two arms and two legs, is manifesting these aspects.

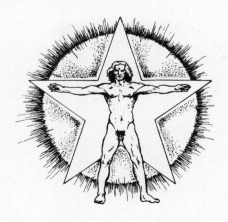

What is experienced looking inwards to the still center can also be seen in the manifestation of outward expression. The Trinity of the spirit within can be seen manifested in nature around us and this is represented in the six-pointed Star of David. The six points of the star could be experienced as the main direction which consciousness may take.

1) Aspiring to a higher level of vibration.
2) Being humble and receptive to new learning.
3) Expressing actively through nature on one's present level.
4) Listening passively to the sound of nature as it is.
5) Looking inwards with introspection and awe.
6) Being aware of all the fine detail of expression with wonder.

Looking at the latter six aspects takes in another aspect and brings us to the SEVEN levels of consciousness.

AN EXPANSION OF THE SEVEN LEVELS OF CONSCIOUSNESS

Up to now in this course we have looked at the seven levels of consciousness in depth and outlined ways of experiencing each level in detail. The evolution of consciousness starts at naught and moves through many changes before returning to naught.

Cycles of growth within growth are taking place. In looking inwards we retrace the steps already taken. In looking outwards we see the growth of those who have gone before us. Purely on the level of matter, atoms have grown to molecules, elements have united to form compounds and, on a planetary scale, solar systems are associating and growing with galactic fusions.

On the level of nature, cells have grown into plant life, animal form, and human consciousness. The future promises a further growth to the global awareness of a Planetary Man, then to the pure light of an elevated state of Universal Being.

The way in which growth takes place on all levels is the challenge of a new situation to come, or a change of circumstances that demand a surrendering effort to a new pattern of living.

The techniques of the growth path we choose and the patterns of life that we design all necessitate the integrated use of the seven levels of consciousness. In using them wisely we are taken inwards to our True Center and brought outwards with a development of our abilities and responsibilities.

The seven main types of posture in Hatha Yoga are Standing, Lying, Inverted, Twisting, Forward-Bending, Back-Bending and Sitting. These positions provide situations which direct the consciousness into the center of a universal vibration (chakra) that is an essential factor for the maintenance of life and the pattern of living necessary for the enlightenment of conscious man.

The needs of a community of people also present seven situations which, when mastered, can create a framework for perfect harmonious living. In meeting the challenges of society, the community as a whole can discover the functions of each of the seven main areas of life and realize the creative spirit in each that will enable the community to live in Truth and expand onto higher levels of existence.

Following is a list of the needs for the maintainance, creativity and responsibility of expanding consciousness. Also the postures that bring awareness of the areas of life that provide these needs.

252

COLOR OF LIGHT	SPIRITUAL DIRECTIVE	NATURE OF MIND	BODY POSITION	ENVIRONMENT
Violet	Visualizing	Imagining	Lying	Art & Presentation
Indigo	Formulating	Idealizing	Sitting	Research & Design
Blue	Synthesizing	Authorizing	Inverted	Government & Religion
Green	Energizing	Securing	Back-Bending	Economics & Finance
Yellow	Analyzing	Questioning	Twisting	Communication & Education
Orange	Integrating	Socializing	Forward-Bending	Relationship & Locality
Red	Establishing	Stabilizing	Standing	Home & Position

DRAWING A MAP OF CONSCIOUSNESS

Consciousness exists on many levels and has many aspects. When we consciously look inwards to a deepening center of our Being, or consciously look outwards to the expanding expression of life, more aspects are revealed, and more areas of consciousness are experienced and a growth in one area is reflected in all areas.

The many aspects of the self provide sign-posts and viewpoints on the map of universal consciousness in which we may site our own individual state and space at any one time. We may also recognize the areas of consciousness in which those around us are operating and thereby see the relationship of each one to the whole, and we may also realize the fact that the same pure consciousness is in all.

On the physical level, we can use the body as a map of consciousness to see the direction and way in which our beam of consciousness needs to 'scan' in order to bring about a perfect balance and proportioning of consciousness. A wobbly leg, a bent spine, or a stiff neck, all need looking into with relationship to the whole body, in order to see where positive and negative energy has fixed itself and needs to flow more freely with true direction.

The mental and spiritual aspects correlating to these defects need also to be examined. The way in which we find it possible to bring the body into alignment and fitness can also be applied on mental and spiritual levels. If, in order to eliminate a stiff neck the shoulder stand is required, what position (attitude) does the mind need to be in to work through a similar rigidity of thought? How open are we to our own inner authority (conscience) and changing emotions, which are the subtler aspects of this particular part of the body?

The fulfillment of our innermost motivations and the lack of them may also be seen on all levels. The direction in which we have come is shown in the habits of behavior and the conditioning that has placed us where we are right now. What we need to insure is that we are taking the most direct road to a state of divine centeredness with the divine order around us.

There are many ways in which we can plot a map of consciousness. The essential requirement to all, however, is an honest looking and studying of our own and others' behavior patterns. Actions, breathing, thinking and feelings are but a few areas in which we can create a situation and then observe and experience the reaction and nature of consciousness. If we examine our approach to life with an openness to change, we can see the possibilities for discovering new "ground" and mastering the old.

Divination is one process of seeing "where we are at", and of seeing the routes to further development that are possible. We can consult an oracle such as the I Ching or look with the Tarot. We can question ourself by using a pendulum, or we can gaze at a spot on the wall and see with direct perception. Because direct perception is difficult to master, the ancient prophets used divining instruments to prevent the subtle energies of the spirit from being swamped by the more gross vibrations we are used to dealing with. Moses and Aaron had rods, Jacob a multicolored divining coat, the ancient Egyptians had the ankh rod and the merkhet pendulum. Christopher Hills wanted to place this powerful technique of tuning into God's will into the hands of everybody. Therefore, he developed a series of pendulums and other divining instruments to specifically select and amplify both the user's divining ability and the subtle vibrations being detected. Hills' main work on divination is in his book *Supersensonics** in which he shows how a master of divination can determine what works for him in any situation and thus be constantly in tune with the Self.

Another map of consciousness that shows the forces that govern our actions and the nature of the universe around us is the zodiac. Astrology can be used to develop our consciousness so that we may govern ourself in closer attunement to the Principal guiding the whole zodiacal configuration of energies in man.

* Supersensonics -- The Science of Consciousness -- is a comprehensive work exploring the nature of consciousness through divination.

Other books Christopher Hills has written on this subject include "Rays From the Capstone" and "Instruments of Knowing" available from the University of the Trees Press, P.O. Box 644, Boulder Creek, CA 95006.

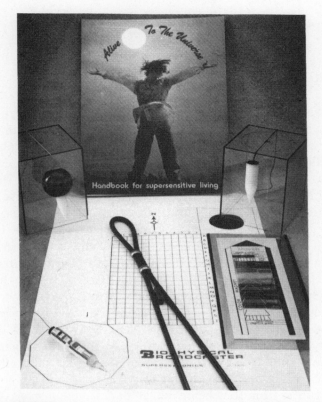

Advanced Assortment
of Divining Instruments*

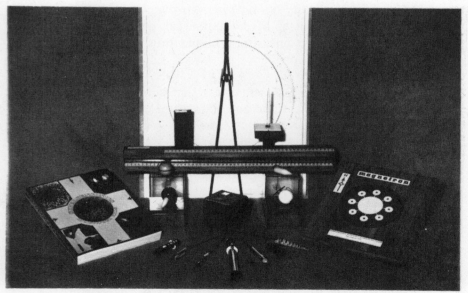

Professional Assortment of Divining and Radionic Instruments*

* For further information write University of the Trees Press, P.O Box 644, Boulder Creek,
Calif. 95006.

The Bible or other great teachings of the masters can also be studied in order to see how the laws of consciousness are guiding us personally towards the Truth. For example, with the consciousness centered on God (the absolute of life), open the Bible ad-lib at any page. If this is done with real sincerity and an openness to learning, on the page that is opened will be the appropriate message for the present situation and state of affairs.

In a similar way, centering the consciousness on a meaningful question and placing the I Ching on the forehead we throw three coins six times. As instructed in the book, we can check this personal interaction with the universe by constructing the appropriate hexagram of forces from the way in which the coins fall. This resulting hexagram is relevant to you at that moment and its reading will be appropriate to your situation at that time.

By studying a section of a teaching that is close to the heart and which we greatly respect, we may also find opportunities for understanding the SELF and life's situations.

Life itself is also a map of consciousness and when studied consciously it can reveal at any moment the laws of the universe and how they are affecting us personally. There are four main directives in life which open up the gateways to Truth. The four aspects of consciousness with which these directives deal are Action, Devotion, Knowledge and Meditation.

What follows is a self-study program that relates the behavior of the world in which we are involved to our own behavior and this, in turn, to the divine pattern of living that emanates from the Center within all living entities. The program is for practicing every moment of the day.

METHOD FOR SELF-KNOWLEDGE

1) Continuously observe and experience consciousness from the viewpoint of looking and listening to the whole field of life energies surrounding a situation.

2) Keep a constant attunement of the individual will with the will of the universe by being honest in seeing both "what is most important and needs to be done", and "what is most relevant to the situation at hand".

3) Study life in terms of the following:

What are you doing? -- What is your "business" in life?

Our job, whether it be Housewife or Engineer, Teacher or Servant, is the means by which we manifest life in order to create, maintain and change the physical structure and environment patterns that shape our society and situation.

On whatever level we place the consciousness, environment, body, breath, mind, etc. this gateway of seeing what we are doing opens up the possibility of increasing consciousness. See:
> What is your potential with consciousness?
> What is being done on each level right now?
> What can be done on all levels?
> What needs to be done?

These are self-encounter questions which can challenge the consciousness to grow.

How do you do what you do? -- How "artistic" is your living?

This devotion aspect lifts and refines what we do onto another level of vibration and gives dimension and form to it.

Language is an example of the way in which a person or nation expresses common situations in life in a different way and so adds a unique quality to the expression of Man as a whole.

How do we walk, communicate, talk, breathe?

Can we discriminate true art from a description of self-indulgence or self-limiting consciousness?

To eat what one drinks and drink what one eats is a Zen example of the way to increase the art of living consciously.

Why do you do what you do? -- How "scientific" is your reasoning?

The motivations of every action provide the self-knowledge aspect which lends meaning to life. It makes it possible to know the cause and effect principle (Law of Karma) in detail. A constant vigilance to see why we do what we do can enable us to recognize the enlightening and delusive forces and why they shape our nature in the way that they do.

Who is doing what you do? -- Who is "Governing" and who is the Authority in your life?

Whether or not we seek guidance from a spiritual master or follow the law of the land, we need to realize our own decision making faculty to the extent that we can see with a non-attached perspective and fulfill the real need of every situation with true consideration for others as ourself.

The offering of what we do to an unknown God, a life Principal or a Unifying force lends a purpose to life and brings action, art and science onto a deeper level of love.

It creates a channel for a greater wisdom to guide our lives.

Who is governing your life right now? Do you look outwards for authority and guidance or do you look inwards to your own conscience and reason? Can you see guidance and the authoritative Truth in your inner and outer worlds?

In bringing all four of the above aspects into our life every moment of the day, action, devotion, knowledge and the self-discipline of Meditation can be brought into a state of Divinity which is a doing without seeking rewards of any kind.

Doing without doing what we do is an effortless state in which it is clearly seen what has to be done and is consciously done with joy in the heart, wisdom in the head and peace in the soul. Living with this love, the Truth of an individual "I" and the Universal Principle as ONE is made real, and the consciousness is purified by a non-attached total involvement in all that is done, which creates interest and wonder in all that is seen.

When there is no disturbance or separation from all that is done and seen, there is an open consciousness of what is being done, how it is being done, and why it is being done. The entry of any ego identifications can soon be seen and removed. The mind attachments can likewise be transcended so that the pure SPIRIT and immortal NATURE of the ONE can be lived with a freedom from structure yet working spontaneously with it.

When one can personalize the impersonal or impersonalize the personal, macrocosms are seen in microcosms and microcosms are seen as a macrocosmic world of ourselves. What is happening in the inner world and the world around us are all reflections of the ONE self in the mirror of life. Look into it and see, for your SELF.

260

PART 14

UNITY THROUGH WHOLENESS

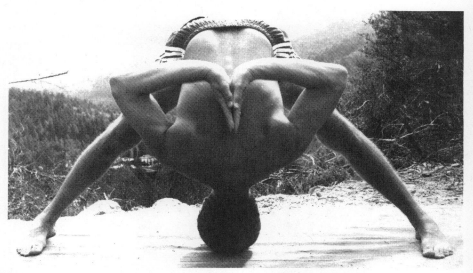

OR

WHOLENESS IN DIVERSITY

PATHS TO ENLIGHTENMENT

From space, the hollow in the womb of the cosmos, nature is born. The original reason why and how the motivating love brought about by conception and birth is never told, perhaps because there is no need. The universe knows its own need and supplies its own need; otherwise, life would not exist. The cosmic spirit of Truth (Heavenly Father) and universal love in the heart of nature (Divine Mother) are eternally united as ONE, evolving through inspiration (Contraction) and aspiration (Expansion). Thus, the cosmic will brings forth its manifestations of creation.

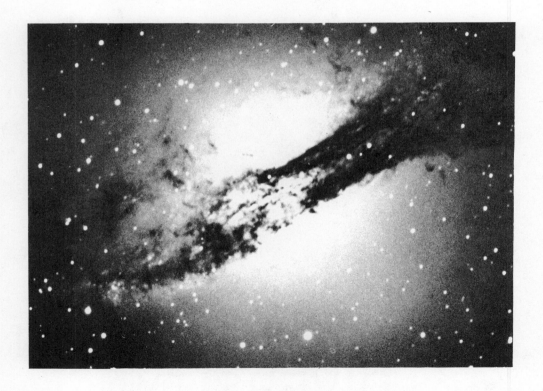

From the central space within each atom of matter, these contractions and expansions are taking place and, from within our own body, energy is constantly being released from the nucleus of each cell as it is caused to contract and expand by the ONE.

Pure spirit sees all as itself and its will is absolute. The projection of this pure consciousness into its image in colored form produces the dualistic state of knowing and a not-knowing self. Awareness and ignorance cause the shaping of all things and, in man, these combine in differing proportions according to his I-identification. When a man sees his all-knowing self (God state or consciousness) and his un-knowing, separated state of falseness, he realizes the reality of the ONE who leads him to a state of pure consciousness enlightened with the conscious unfoldment of the whole SELF and the development of consciousness according to divine law.

Although it may sometimes seem that consciousness and life can be "wrapped up in a nutshell", God is ever presenting himself with new problems, new designs and new ways of looking at himself. Whenever one feels smug, proud, or thinks he knows himself, God presents another picture of life at which to look and discover Truth anew.

It is God's perogative to re-create; it is the need of consciousness to experience it. Though one must learn to rise above experience, one must be prepared to go deep into it, if necessary. The passion of Jesus Christ and the compassion of the Buddha teach us this. There are others, too, who have transcended experience, and yet have been able to show their love of the Divine by a sacrifice of human values for superhuman manifestations for a giving to the world for the sake of the ONENESS in all things. The attitudes and ways of these masters offer paths to the enlightened state which they have attained.

Enlightenment is the state of awareness that leaves no doubt in a person that he and the Godhead and the Life Force in all things are as one, and that his real existence is immortality.

One who is "On the Path" to enlightenment is one who is consciously seeking to reach this state of awareness through an ever increasing and deepening experience of life and of knowing in terms of Self-realization.

Is there more than one path?

There are some things in life which are definable in words and some things which are not. We can talk about something in such a way that it may stimulate an interest in the listener to experience it for himself. We can even give techniques that may aid the direct experience of what is being talked about. The rest is up to the listener and the communication ability of the speaker. The way a person listens, the way a person speaks, the way each person uses his gift of consciousness in expression and introspection, is unique to the individual. Hence, there are ultimately as many paths as there are life entities. There is, however, a common factor called "consciousness" or "being", and the laws by which consciousness in its pure state creates itself, maintains itself and dissolves itself back into a void of stillness, enables man to see the great wonders of the spirit within his own conscious self and in the life that he leads. In this sense there is only one path -- the path of knowing the SELF.

The Common Links

Life cries out that ALL IS ONE and science emphasizes this with an ever increasing number of facts about a universal energy that is formed into the multitudinous patterns of matter, mind stuff and spirit.* What first

* For a deep study of how the universal field manifests itself, see "Supersensonics: the Spiritual Physics of all Vibrations from Zero to Infinity", published by University of the Trees Press.

created this energy is not known. However, it has certain characteristics that can be seen and understood both objectively and subjectively in human terms. For example:

a) Energy exists as a vibration polarized positive and negative and sensed as a physical, mental or spiritual experience through the effects of resonance and harmony.

b) The propagation of energy is through a process of expansion and contraction as in the act of breathing, whether it be in the body or in nature's cycle of day and night, or season come season.

c) The effect of vibrating life energy is to create spirals of evolution and involution, experienced throughout life as growth.

The way in which the above characteristics reflect the purpose and functions of life and guide us to a fulfillment and peace in Self-realization is the subject of this section. Look at the way in which you already experience life now and examine how it relates to the "essence" in the light of the information given. Listen to what is being spoken in terms which are valid for you. Please do not be confused by the different words, symbols, sounds or techniques which follow, but rather open up to the "variations on the theme of life" and discover your own spontaneous melody line in the same key.

Keynote

Whether or not you are convinced that a Godhead or a state of total awareness is within you and behind all creation, what is important is for each one to challenge his own consciousness by acts of faith and self-surrender. Throughout the ages there have been those who have spoken of their inner realizations of the "ONE" and have demonstrated their close relationship to it by a giving of themselves to a remarkable degree. It is to those enlightened ones that others have been compelled to follow certain practices which have enabled them to see that which is beyond what is seen, and to hear what is behind that which is heard. Scientifically speaking, it is interesting to note how all things are affected by a greater force than its conscious self. Whatever moves the whole universe which we see with our consciousness on a macrocosmic level allows us to live in it by the very nature of its existence. At the same time, some Life Principal in our consciousness is allowing the cells and atoms of our own body to exist on a microcosmic level and determine whether or not the heart should beat and the lungs should take another breath of air.

Energy is neither created nor destroyed; IT simply IS. Man's body, mind and spirit consist of energy vibrating at different rates. Consciousness can limit this energy or make it unlimited and the awareness of it can be as simple or complicated as man wishes to make it.

In simple terms, energy flows and vibrates according to polarity, positive/negative, male/female. These forces are drawn together, separated or controlled by the use of a third dimension. In electricity this third dimension is the neutral or earth line.

In the consciousness of man it is the self-sense which focuses or separates what is "liked" and "not liked" through the mind and ego. In the interaction of polarities an over projection causes confusion and pain. Then comes delusion about the true reality of life. A misuse of the mind also brings suffering and ignorance. To break through this self-delusion, there are religious cultures, sciences and all manner of spiritual teachings. Let us now look at the four major gateways to enlightenment, namely, action (Tibetan Yoga), Meditation (Christian Mysticism), Knowledge (Modern Psychology), and Devotion (Eastern Religion).

In these paths considered, all look with awe and wonder to the possible state of liberation from delusion and the freedom from attachment to creation, to a state of consciousness, without need of qualification, since it is pure and complete in itself, its self being the "ALL-ONE" (ALONE).

Diagram 14.1.

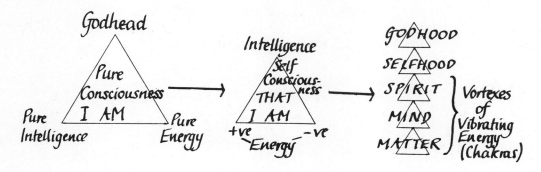

The diagram above depicts the differentiation of this pure consciousness into the state of I AM and the polarity of THIS and THAT, and then further differentiation into spiritual, mental and physical identifications of soul, mind and body. These are ranges of vibration which can be differentiated still further and all are in themselves polarized vortexes of energy which can consciously radiate an electro-magnetic field or aura of individuality such as I AM a MAN, or I AM a HOUSEWIFE, etc.

The aim of giving brief outlines of the "paths" to enlightenment is to help you to guide your consciousness back to its source by letting go of identifications, projections, assumptions and egocentricities that may have been invested in you by these traditional approaches, and to re-establish your true identity which is immortal and beyond all these things, all things being in self-consciousness. Let us now step through the four gateways to enlightenment by putting ourselves into the consciousness of the successors of these paths who, likewise, went beyond method and ritual.

TIBETAN YOGA

Tibetan Yoga could be described as a mixture of the traditional yogas of body (Hatha), mind (Laya), and soul (Raja), and the Tantra Yoga of Buddhism.

The traditional yogas are grouped as follows:

Body control -- Hatha Yoga, incorporating:
  Pranayam -- breath control,
  Padmasan -- the perfection of the lotus posture.

Mind control -- Laya Yoga, incorporating:
  Bhakti Yoga -- devotion to the Supreme one using powers of love.
  Mantra Yoga -- control of sound currents using chanting, word repetition, etc.
  Yantra Yoga -- control of form using symbols and geometrical patterns.

Thought power -- Dhyana Yoga, incorporating:
  Thought processing and mind expansion using Mandalas as a Yidam (teacher).

Self-knowledge -- Raja Yoga, incorporating:
  Jnana Yoga -- divine wisdom, intellectual discrimination.
  Karma Yoga -- right action.
  Kundalini Yoga -- control of psychic powers.
  Samadhi Yoga -- bliss and the control of ecstasy.
  Nirvana Yoga -- total awareness whilst absorbed in bliss.

All the above are practiced in the Tantric Yoga of Tibetan Buddhism. For Tibetans, the need for liberation and devotion to those who have attained it has long influenced their actions in everyday life. Tantra means

268

act or ritual. Given readily to natural expression, the Tibetans describe their act of "Union with the Divine" (the meaning of the word Yoga) in symbols and paintings, clearly defined by their primitive existence. Hence, figures in sexual embrace, a very natural human act of union, are used frequently to depict the blissful union of man with his spiritual essence, as well as male and female aspects of his nature. Tibetan Buddhist Yoga is often referred to as the Yoga of the Great Symbol. The symbol being that symbol which represents a balancing of polarities towards a state of perfection, of liberation, of enlightenment. Examples of this are:

The Dorje -- This is a metal object which is used to meditate upon until the meditator perfects the balance of his own energies and realizes the nature of his centered Self and the power that emanates from it. This power is called the "Vajra" power.

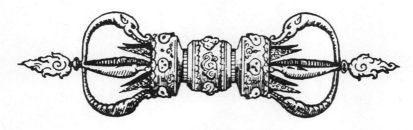

TIBETAN DORJE
SYMBOL OF THE EIGHT LEVELS

The Lotus Posture -- Again, a perfect position of balance in which the Kundalini energy at the base of the spine is stimulated and drawn inwards and up the spine. The centers of wisdom and awareness are awakened by a stimulation of the brain cells and glands in the head.

The Chant OM MANI PADME HUM -- These words mean "The Absolute One, creating, maintaining and dissolving into bliss, is the jewel in the heart of the Lotus, and is none other than my True Self."

The lotus flower unfolds its pure white leaves from out of the muddy waters in which it grows. Whatever state our consciousness is in now, we too can unfold that Pure Consciousness that is lying dormant within. Hence, constant repetition, contemplation and absorption in the chanting of this mantra, can eventually bring forth the pure state of Nirvana (enlightenment).

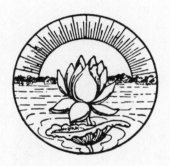

The above incorporate techniques that help the aspirant to concentrate and meditate upon the true nature of his existence. All aspects of his being are seen as he goes towards his goal, and the mastering of the various energies and states of consciousness are depicted and enhanced by Mandalas (maps of consciousness), Yantras (fixation patterns), Thankas (paintings on cloth), and the various Buddhas (Godlike Beings) that remind the meditator of those who, in physical form, have attained that which he seeks.

The Iconography of the maps of consciousness expressed in Tibetan art reveals the "common links" in our study into consciousness. Note the basic patterns in the Divine Structure outlined and in the pictures which follow.

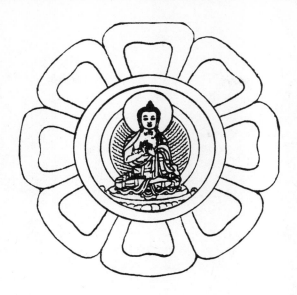

Diagram 14.2.

BUDDHA
Divine Body
Perfect form of human being
The essential One

TRI-KAYA
(Triple Gem)

SAMBHOGA
Divine body of people on the
path. Buddhas and Bodisatt-
vas who have postponed
entry into Nirvana in order
to free unenlightened ones.
The Reflected One.

DHARMA
Divine body of Truth, work-
ing out the wheel of life.
The practical aspect.

DHYANI BUDDHAS
Unmanifested spirit of various
attributes.

DHYANI BODHISATTVAS
Manifested qualities of Dhyani Buddhas.

ELEMENTS

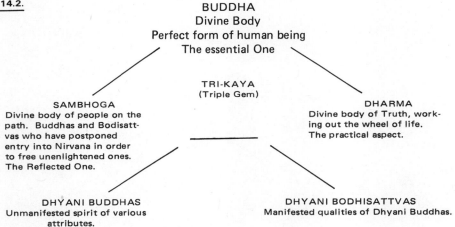

VAIROCANA -- The Absolute	ether	SAMATABHADRA -- Universal kindness
AMOGHASIDDHI -- Volition	air	VISVAPANI --
VAIROCANA -- The Absolute	ether	SAMATABHADRA -- Universal kindness
AMOGHASIDDHI -- Volition	air	VISVAPANI -- All-perceptive light
AMITABHA -- Perception	fire	AVOLOKITA -- Compassion
AKSOBHYA -- Form	water	VAJRAPANI -- Supreme power
RATNASAMBHAVA -- Feeling (matter)	earth	RATNAPANI -- Wisdom of equality

271

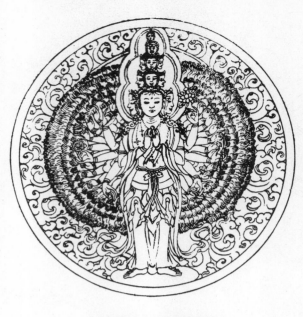

AVALOKITESHVARA

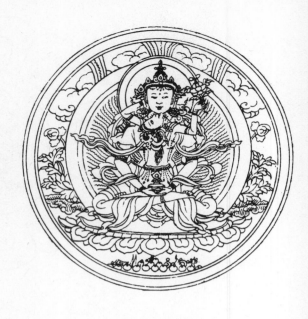

ADI BUDDHA

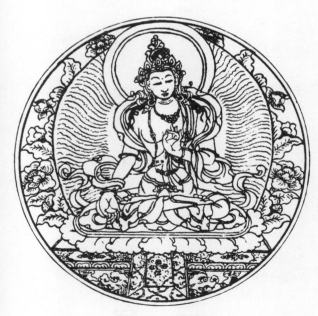

SHAKYAMUNI

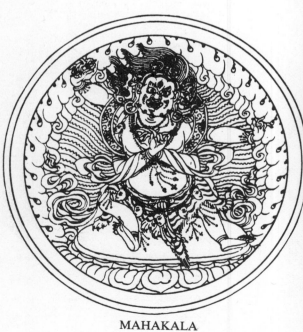

MAHAKALA

272

In paintings the Boddhisattvas are shown with three heads (the three forces of nature: positive, negative, neutral), and five levels of three heads depict the three forces of nature acting through the five chakras. In Tibetan Yoga the top two chakras and the bottom two chakras of the traditional yoga system are as one. Some paintings show aspects of mercy, as in the green Goddess Tara, or of enlightenment as in the Adi Buddha. Others, like Maha Kala, show the fearlessness that is needed to stamp out the undesirable temptations of the ego (note figure of man under the foot). Other aspects may not be seen clearly until many months or even years of meditation on a mandala have been practiced. On the other hand, you may see them in the next second and recognize the self who has identified with it.

The result of all effort is shown in the manifestation of the person making it. When one meets Tibetans and sees them at their work one cannot help but notice their unusually bright eyes and keen sense of perception. They are extremely practical as well as esoteric, and their devotion is carried with them throughout the day in the form of a prayer wheel or other reminder of their love for the Buddhahood. The three Lokas or evils which they aim to avoid are anger, sloth and passion. They replace these with affection, love and compassion. Gautama, the manifested Buddha, emphasizes compassionate service to mankind and love for the Buddhahood, together with those on the path. Yoga is the means to attaining this and it is practiced faithfully by Lamas and householders alike. As with all things, the true experience comes through involvement and practice to the extent of complete absorption and loss of self-consciousness. The result is NIRVANA, the goal of Tibetan Yoga.

CHRISTIAN MYSTICISM

What is mystery to one person may be clear to another. In fact it may be that the mystery is in communicating what is perfectly natural to someone who is on another level of experience. If a person of what we call normal education were to take a transistor radio into the jungle and present it to a tribe of natives, it would be very difficult to describe what it is and how it works in terms of radio waves and the theory of electricity in order that the natives could understand. One would probably have to use the language of the tribe and call it the God of sound who can make different sounds with different tongues when you turn this ear or nose, according to where the controls are on the radio set. With a good education those natives could eventually appreciate the music that is coming out of the set and know how and why it works the way it does.

In mysticism, experiences are often expressed in words clothed in symbolism and which have no meaning and relevance to the uninitiated. However, they may stimulate the imagination and the desire to understand what is being communicated. To experience what St. John in Revelations calls "the sound of a trumpet" and the vision of "seven candlesticks" and "seven stars", one has to be in a certain state of readiness on the spiritual path. In order to receive the teachings and see the vision that is being related may take many years of meditation and introspection.

In the introduction we talked about an all-pervading energy. This energy is vibrating and can be heard in moments of silence and inner stillness. This is the trumpet sound referred to by St. John. It is also the Word of God referred to in Genesis. Again in Genesis it talks about a firmament. This is the space between the unmanifested and manifested states of consciousness, i.e. the Pure Conscious state in which the all-knowing intelligence (Christ Consciousness) resides. The waters are the elements earth, water, fire, air, and ether in their unmanifested form.

When St. John talks about the seven candlesticks, he is referring to the seven chakras, the vortexes of energy out of which the seven spirits (elemental energies above) manifest as seven energy centers (stars) in the body. The centers can be seen inwardly on the astral level of consciousness as lights. The areas of the body which develop from this light energy are the seven major parts (legs, stomach, heart, etc.) which St. John related to as the seven churches. He calls polarity "a two-edged sword".

The "common" link in Christian Mysticism with the framework of consciousness given in the introduction is shown below.

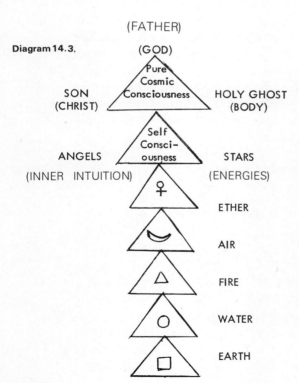

Diagram 14.3.

(FATHER)
(GOD)

SON (CHRIST)

ANGELS
(INNER INTUITION)

HOLY GHOST (BODY)

STARS
(ENERGIES)

Pure Cosmic Consciousness

Self Consciousness

ETHER

AIR

FIRE

WATER

EARTH

Anyone can experience these things by developing his perception and "inner world" of consciousness.

Ascetics of the Christian religion follow the teachings of the manifested Christ embodied in the perfection found in the bodily form of Jesus.

Jesus taught a life of non-attachment which is attainable wherever you are. However, in order to concentrate uninterruptedly, certain ascetics and Christian saints have led a life of seclusion and austerity.

275

Through long periods of meditation and prayer, mystics draw themselves closer to that inner, Christ-like state of consciousness. They may choose to manifest this radiance in seclusion on a spiritual level that most humans are not even aware of in themselves. On the other hand, they may share it on the physical plane. Rejection of life on any level never brings true godliness since life was made to be lived. Accepting others as they are, being firm and steady in one's own path, and serving others through a sharing of the life energy, on whatever level, is the true way. Saints like St. Francis, Thomas A. Kempis, and the early apostles, were all men of compassion and understanding, though with themselves they were ruthless enough to not be distracted by the whims of the senses or the need for ego satisfaction. Either through long periods of praying in one position or in devotion to work, like St. Francis in the kitchen, Christian mystics have found their way to God and have understood the nature of consciousness.

The life of a Christian mystic is told in the book *The Way of a Pilgrim*. By total absorption in the prayer "Lord Jesus Christ have mercy on me" the mystic is taken into many experiences in life in which he is tested with endurance and hardship, but rewarded with a constant feeling of the presence of God and an understanding of the life he has been given.

Rituals, Techniques and Symbols

The mystical union of human consciousness with the Christ-conscious state is ritualized in the act of Holy Communion, in which bread as the symbol of energy, and water as the symbol of spontaneous intelligence, are taken. With the communion of self-effort (energy) and the development of awareness (intelligence), one is made ready to receive the true UNION of man with his creator.

This union is symbolized in the sign of the cross. When spirit (the all-knowing Christ aspect) is brought into nature (the all-present aspect), and nature (referred to as the Holy Ghost) is given up to spirit, then Man becomes whole (Holy).

Diagram 14.4.

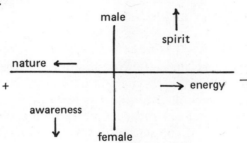

A balance of these aspects brings the at-one-ment (atonement) with the Father (Creator). This state can be attained by prayer and fasting, that is, a letting go of the delusion that the body is the only existence. Also, by meditation on the meaning of the cross and the words of Jesus the Truth is realized in oneself. Only by the total sacrifice of selfishness or the complete faith in God can the union be lasting. That union cannot be described and hence it is mysterious. Mystics search for this union within themselves, not by worshiping the actual physical body of Jesus, or feeling remorse at his having left the Earth. His willingness to let go of the physical body showed his powerful inner strength that he used selflessly in allowing himself to be crucified. His mastery over delusion through self-effort is the example for others to follow.

What is within a person is eventually manifested and can be seen. In the words of an unnamed Christian mystic, "The depth of a person's meditation can be seen by how much he is aware of who needs the salt and pepper at the dinner table and how willing he is to dig the garden when it needs doing without being asked."

MODERN PSYCHOLOGY

What is Self and what is not Self? What is the Person and what is the Personality? What is Real and Integrating life; what is unreal and separating it? What do the physiological characteristics of Man mean in terms of mind experience? Who is the "I" that experiences and observes? Who am I?

These are the questions the psychologist might ask as he encounters himself with himself in confrontation with others and with life's situations. The breaking down of psychological barriers to find a more integrated being has led such people as Jung and Maslow to study the world of sensation and mind experience in order to go beyond it, exploring it and learning how to master it along the way.

Life is an extension of the Self and reflects the light or awareness that is put into it. Think of a beautiful scene, concentrate on it, and sooner or later that scene will be experienced in the world of the senses, for we see with consciousness and consciousness is what is seen. Matter is born out of a concentration of vibrating light energy. Under pressure and temperature change, light fuses into the elements that vibrate to form a material substance. Consciousness itself is a superfine vibration which condenses into light under certain conditions. Continue to pressurize and heat matter and it eventually turns back into light and then consciousness. Such is the ability of consciousness to focus into itself.

THE FOCUSING OF CONSCIOUSNESS

The light of consciousness (awareness) is focused in the same way that light is focused through a lens. The diagram below is a repeat of an earlier drawing in Section 1.

Diagram 14.5.

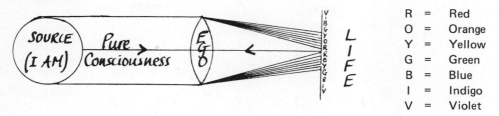

R = Red
O = Orange
Y = Yellow
G = Green
B = Blue
I = Indigo
V = Violet

Certain western psychologists such as Dr. Max Luscher and Dr. Christopher Hills have shown that there is a direct correlation between color, the personality and consciousness. In his book *Nuclear Evolution: Discovery of the Rainbow Body* Christopher Hills explains how evolution comes through a clear seeing of the effects of positive and negative charge on each level of vibration as shown in diagram 14.6 and the ability to change by expansion and refinement of the personality. This process of change produces changes in the electro-magnetic aura of the person and of his environment. A person can also absorb into his aura the vibrations from color in his environment, which in turn can affect the nature of the person and change his auric vibrations.

The diagram 14.6 shows the various levels of consciousness and the color of the aura which they produce. Like layers of an onion, they can be peeled off to reveal the no-thingness of self-annihilation (freedom from identification). The levels can also be balanced to produce a total integration into pure light.

In the movement of consciousness indicated by the arrows, negative and positive energies spiral inwards and outwards, expanding and contracting according to relationship and identification.

Diagram 14.6.

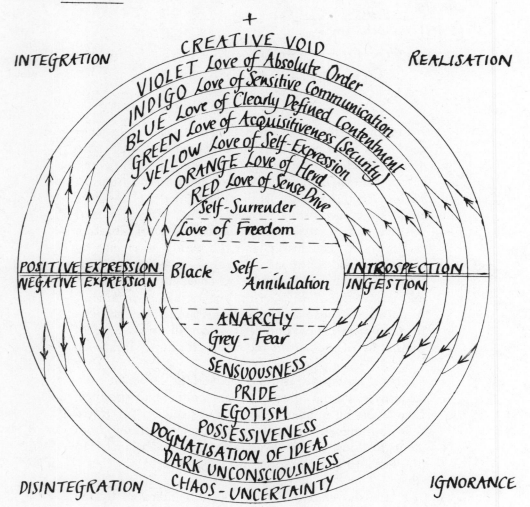

INTEGRATION

REALISATION

+

CREATIVE VOID

VIOLET Love of Absolute Order

INDIGO Love of Sensitive Communication

BLUE Love of Clearly Defined Contentment

GREEN Love of Acquisitiveness (Security)

YELLOW Love of Self-Expression

ORANGE Love of Herd

RED Love of Sense Drive

Self-Surrender

Love of Freedom

POSITIVE EXPRESSION

NEGATIVE EXPRESSION

Black   Self-Annihilation

INTROSPECTION

INGESTION

ANARCHY

Grey - Fear

SENSUOUSNESS

PRIDE

EGOTISM

POSSESSIVENESS

DOGMATISATION OF IDEAS

DARK UNCONSCIOUSNESS

CHAOS - UNCERTAINTY

DISINTEGRATION

IGNORANCE

—

The preceding diagrams can be combined and shown as a projection of polarity in triangular force form on relative levels of vibration.

Diagram 14.7.

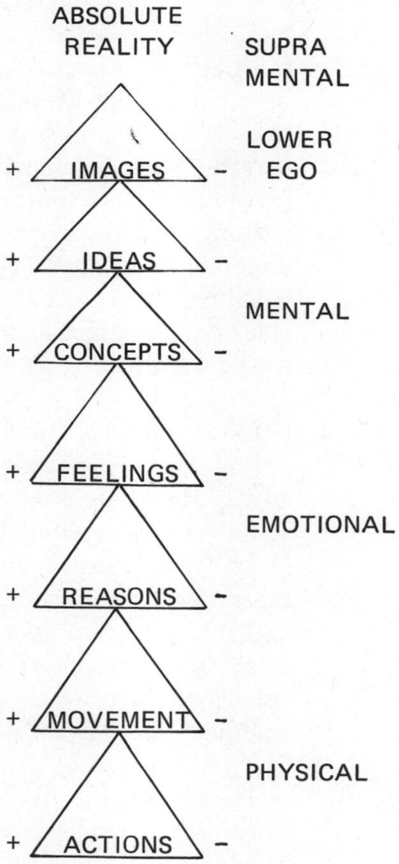

Note again the similarity to our diagram in the introduction.

Here there are seven levels formed from some Absolute "I" force which projects, identifies and associates, according to the degree of awareness.

Through psychology, the breaking down of the barriers that separate us from others and our true Self is a breaking down of the conditioned personality and communication gaps so that all parts of our self can be seen as they really are and used effectively in life.

ABSOLUTE
REALITY   SUPRA
                       MENTAL

SUPER   LOWER
EGO+   + IMAGES -   EGO

           + IDEAS   -
                          MENTAL
           + CONCEPTS -

           + FEELINGS -
                          EMOTIONAL
           + REASONS   -

           + MOVEMENT -
                          PHYSICAL
           + ACTIONS   -

281

Techniques

Gestalt therapy, often used nowadays by fringe psychologists and encounter groups, uses techniques such as "primal scream" in which inhibitions are allowed to be expressed by screaming and groaning. Also, encounter situations are used, such as looking a person in the eyes and saying exactly what you see in him and feel about him, and vice versa. Violence is not allowed and reactions are examined. An intelligent study of who is the "I" that screams, sees and feels is the aim, together with the "I" that thinks, does and imagines. The outcome may be positive characterstics or negative traits. There may also be ego patterns of consciousness or universal patterns which have a definite purpose in creating and understanding the ONE who is creating and understanding. The skill in encounter work comes from the ability to be open and to change to what is appropriate to the situation.

Often eastern thinking, yoga and meditation techniques are used to process the mind onto a supra-mental level. Hypnosis is another technique which has taken some people seemingly back into past incarnations. Deep trance states can be useful for relaxing a person prior to questioning him about experiences he is having and the subconscious motives behind his actions. Electroencephalographs (E.E.G. machines) and relaxometers are also used to see the effect of brain wave patterns and responses to states of depravation.

The effects of color, sound and personal contact can cause a resonance experienced as a harmonious feeling of liking and agreeing in the consciousness. They can also cause a dissonance and nauseating effect. Both can be used to examine and challenge a person to look at himself, for what we see and experience with our senses, whether it be in others or ourselves, is in reality seen with our mind and translated into terms of truth by our own consciousness. There is no other than the Self, yet that Self is very big. It is also smaller than the minutest particle.

To follow the way of modern psychology you say what you mind but mind what you say. Ask why? What said it? Who said it? How was it said? In action you may find yourself motivated by the words of the Gestalt prayer:

You do what you do and I do what I do.
If your thing and my thing are the same thing,
    that's O.K.
If your thing is not my thing, that's O.K. too.
You do what you do and I do what I do.

AMEN.

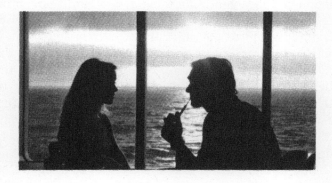

EASTERN RELIGIONS

The path of devotion to an unknown God personified in some human being is common to Islam, Sikh, Hinduism and Christianity (originally an Eastern religion) and it is probably the easiest path to understand from a Westerner's point of view. Less easy to understand, perhaps, is the devotion to some non-imaginative state of perfection common to the Zen Buddhism of Japan and the Taoism of China.

The fact of feeling a presence of some God or Godlike state of consciousness beyond normal human comprehension has been felt by many people at some time or other. Whether or not it has been acknowledged is another matter. More important is the question: has it been a continuous process that has brought about an evolution of the consciousness? True devotion to the "ONE" or "ONENESS" brings a response that gives a greater inner security, an ability to manifest creatively, and a wisdom that cannot be learned from books. True religion is a means of reminding us and confirming in us our duty to that which we acknowledge as Truth. It uses ritual and scriptures as guidelines to attaining a oneness that the writers of the scriptures and the founders of the religions attained. Please note that the founders of the religions found their God outside the orthodoxy of religion. Religion is a man-made practice like a technique. Devotion goes beyond religion and unites man's heart with the heart of life itself. This has no bounds, labels or definable likes or dislikes. To limit God in any way and say God is this or God is that only creates a separation from him. The God that exists in all things can be seen reflected in all things and his ways are universal. These ways show the effects of his presence and describe his nature, but who can really describe that which is creating the very consciousness that is describing? Who can know that which he does not know?

In Zen, the study of such questions as "How does water hold water?" and "How does a knife cut itself?" are a means to understanding the riddle of life. A young monk may spend years looking into the essence of his Koan. A Koan such as "Listen to the sound of one hand clapping" can, if truly meditated upon, bring one to the point of enlightenment in which no sound and all sound is heard.

In Taoism, paradoxes such as "Be empty and be full", "Bend and be straight", are studied with devotion until there is a realization that polarity is an ever-changing and exchanging process of the one Life Principle. Know the Principle, and you know when right turns into wrong and wrong turns into right. All things, when pursued to the ultimate end, turn into their opposite.

The symbol of Yin (ingoing energy) and Yang (outward expression) is shown below. Meditate upon it, feeling its symmetry and significance. The ability to "Go with the flow" is much stressed in Far Eastern culture. Nature provides the reflection of Truth and man must follow the seasons and the signs of the times for attunement to the WISE ONE.

Diagram 14.8.

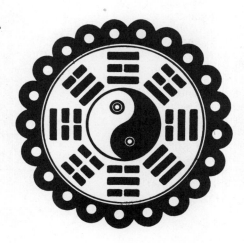

285

Every religion has its own "Bible". For Hindus the Bhagavad Gita relates man's inner struggle in turning to the ways of his creator through the story of a relationship between Krishna, a prince, and Arjuna, his disciple. The physical situations reflect the inner conditions of man's consciousness --- the Guru within and the lower self.

Whether it be the Koran of the Mohammedan, the Bible of the Christian, or the Bhagavad Gita of the Hindu, all present the Truth for those who have "eyes to see and ears to hear". In India, Brahman is the name for God, the creator, together with Vishnu, the maintainer, and Shiva, the destroyer. Here again is the triune of three major powers of God-consciousness. To the Hindu life is a process of overcoming the delusion (maya) caused by these three forces as they manifest in aspects of Shiva/Shakti (Male/Female), and Purusa/Prakriti (impersonal/personal). The diagram following shows this in triangular form with the all-pervading AUM sound emanating from the primal forces.

Diagram 14.9.

Deities are used to denote aspects of the different levels of consciousness. God is often worshipped in the form of the Divine Mother. The Goddess of Death, Kali, is like Maha Kala in the Buddhist religion, the ferocious state of consciousness that puts death to the ego and sense distractions. Ganesh, the Elephant God, is the Deity of Wisdom.

All forms are reflections of aspects of the worshipper, and he worships not the idol but, with concentration and attention, draws to himself the aspect it is portraying.

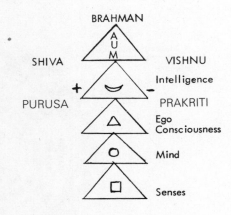

Techniques

Prayer is the most well known of all devotional techniques, if such a word could be used. A simple, sincere prayer from the heart creates a psychic vacuum in the consciousness which draws to it that which is asked. With it comes the responsibility and the comfort of feeling that somehow there is a God who is close enough to know our real needs.

Chanting is another well known means of invoking God's presence and, at the same time, expressing love in a physical way.

Ritual -- The tapping of bells, banging of gongs, and all the ritualistic ceremonies of worship and service can, with the right attitude in the consciousness, affect change by diverting negative forces and attracting positive forces into one's life. A candle flame has the property of keeping at bay psychic disturbances. Visualizing rays of white light and imaging saintly people can have a very positive effect. Incense is a reminder of the purifying effect of the essence within.

The devotion of both the intellectual and the heart-orientated devotee increases his concentration towards the same unknown Force which can be recognized and felt in a personal or impersonal way. Nevertheless, the ultimate experience can never bring forth a description that transmits the actual experience. Lao Tzu puts it in the Tao-Te-Ching thus:

The Tao that is told is not the eternal Tao.
The name that can be named is not the eternal name.
The nameless is the beginning of heaven and earth.
The named is mother of ten thousand things.
Ever desireless, one can see the mystery.
Ever desiring, one can see the manifestations.
These two spring from the same source
  but differ in name.
This appears as darkness.
Darkness within darkness.
The gate to all mystery.

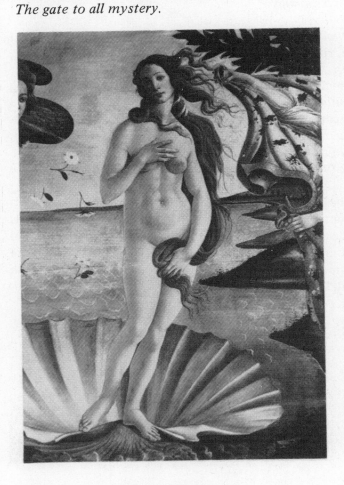

PART 15

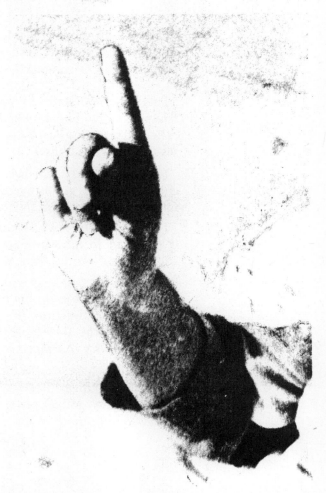

LIVING IN UNION WITH THE HOLY ONE.

THE FACTS OF LIFE

A SUMMARY OF THE PATHS TO TRUTH

The essence of previous descriptions on Tibetan Yoga, Christian Mysticism, Modern Psychology and Eastern Religions can be summarized as follows:

There is *one* state of perfection or Godhead from which all came and to which all eventually turn. This is reflected in life as *unity* and can be seen by one who sees all things as himself.

There is *polarity* which is reflected in life as *diversity* and can be seen as positive and/or negative, according to the point of view of the seer.

There is a *trinity* which holds all things together. This is reflected in the way nature finds an equilibrium and stability and can be seen in one's *ability to balance* and *to be balanced.*

There is *vibration on many levels,* each having its own purpose and function in the life process. These are reflected in the *variety of life* and can be experienced with the *ability to change.*

All is one which is reflected in the *universal laws* which apply to all things. These can be observed in one's own consciousness and experienced totally when one sees *oneself in all things.*

Diagram 15.1.

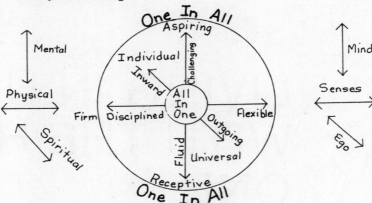

290

THE WAY AHEAD

As the Age of Pisces moves into the Age of Aquarius, there comes a new dawning, an awakening. Uranus rules Aquarius and brings with it a transformation of the old to the new amongst all those who will allow for the change that is required. The integrating of what has gone before into an understanding of the many cycles of our evolution up to the present time prepares the way for new things to come and new horizons to be challenged. The expansion of consciousness does not mean a rejection of what has already been, nor does it mean that we live on "Cloud Nine". There is that which is eternal and that which is changing and both have their place in all universal patterns. The existence of matter is a fact of life just as much as the ability of spirit to create it is a potential energy that is ever present. Wherever there is a vibration of energy there is polarity and this, too, is a fact of life. The ability of consciousness to separate itself and to reintegrate itself is a healthy state, for evolution can then take its course more freely and with a more certain direction.

THE NEW AGE PATH

The coming New Age will teach us how to change more willingly yet be humble to the greater forces within our consciousness that know the way and can guide us along "The Path". We can assist this whole process of evolution by making ourselves more adaptable and more flexible to the true need of the moment. At the same time, there is need to balance this with the following of what one sees to be true, with discipline and firmness. Together these create a growing process based on wisdom and a love of the Source that created all things, so that we may know our Self and look with awe and wonder at the possibilities that life holds in store for us.

An acknowledgement of the Source and a unified field of varying life energy is our prime consideration for a true, integrated and harmonious life. The sharing of life's essence with others, consciously or unconsciously, that they may see it in themselves, is the glue that creates an unparalleled bond of unity. Worship like a Hindu, think like a modern psychologist, act like a yogi, and "know thyself" as in meditation. All paths lead to the one goal and just as by knowing the many roads that go to a certain destination you can choose the most appropriate, so a knowing of the most suitable path can ensure a successful journey.

Paths and the techniques they present can enable you to go as you will towards the state of enlightenment. However, beware! Enlightenment is not attainable by technique alone, and dilly-dallying on the way can lead one "up the garden path". Find the most direct yet practical route for you and follow it closely. Once in the state of enlightenment you have the choice and opportunity to take other routes. Without enlightenment you are a slave to destiny and chance. Love, practice, wisdom and a skill in operation, are all necessary and, therefore, it is useful to develop them by examining the methods and results of those who have gone before. All that is needed is in the eternal now, and it is provided if we look and listen with openness and love. Take one step forward toward God and he takes two steps to meet you.

If you take the prayer of the Mystic and ask with sincerity in the heart "Christ come into my heart and show me how to live my life your way", he will come.

If you sit patiently in the lotus posture of the Yogi and wait in the stillness of your own soul, letting all thoughts disappear, he will come.

If you study every psychological experience to its roots and ask relentlessly "Who am I", allowing no separation between you and the world you observe, he will come.

If you live religiously by the laws of the universe as they unfold themselves to you and make every moment in thought, feeling and action, an offering to the One without a second thought, and without expectation of reward, he will come.

FREEDOM WITH STRUCTURE

The nature of SPIRIT is to freely create structures and to change them with intelligence and direction to a new order of TRUTH in accordance with the reality of nature.

The spirit of NATURE is to move freely with the structure in which it finds itself, expanding it by its own fulfillment in the expression of TRUTH and with an understanding of the order of things.

The influence on structure and movement comes from the ONE source that is still, yet embraces both spirit and nature in its guiding of the vibratory patterns that emerge from it both in spirit and in nature.

Out of this TRINITY of TRUTH, SPIRIT and NATURE matter is born in consciousness by consciousness. With soul, mind, body, environmental and universal energies, consciousness is ever raising, expanding and reflecting back into itself the nature of spirit, the spirit of nature and the presence of the One who is observing and experiencing consciousness as a whole.

Consciousness is what we see with and it is what is seen. With no separation and without attachment to any one thing consciousness is pure.

With this positive state of "no-thing" all parts of the SELF evolve to a new dimension. Without a reference to the positive still center within oneself, a distortion of Truth can occur and then the evolution of both spirit and nature is retarded.

In a society or community, a well-designed structure based on an understanding of the nature of consciousness provides a firm foundation with the means for nature to grow in stature.

Nature provides the flow of energy. When this follows the direction in which it is truly guided, it brings maturity and form to the structure, making it rich and ripe for a change to a state of new responsibilities in the universal pattern of evolution.

Change in itself is meaningless unless it is directed to a higher purpose that can expand its present limits. Expansion is hollow without the support of true direction and real devotion. Direction is inadequate without subjective resourcefulness and a variety in its natural expression of Truth.

Acknowledgement of the ONE controlling and allowing both to take place is the necessary hallowing of the pure vibration that makes life divine. The sincerity of it can be seen manifested by the wise use of shape, energy and form, and by the willingness to make effort, simply in order that evolution may take place at the appointed time.

Any structure can be made to present the necessary challenge of self-discipline for the conscious growth of awareness and ability. Any flow of energy can be spontaneously increased by a constant opening to the inner joy of moving consciousness. Any manifestation can be raised to a higher level of vibration by the sense of balance in positive movement and a deepening of inner calm.

With a person who is self-disciplined to Truth comes the ability to be spontaneous in changing form and structure.

With the person who has a natural flow of energy attuned to Truth will come an ease of spontaneity within any structure.

Every situation can be used to heighten the state of consciousness.

The spirit of truthfulness and sincerity in facing the challenge of an inner structure is seen by refinement and humility.

The effectiveness of a radiant inner joy from spontaneous natural movement is seen in the vibrancy and continuous flow of life energy, shining forth from those who are living consciously in time with the divine spark of life.

A society, a community or any style of living is a structure created by consciousness and can be used for the benefit of its evolution.* It affords situations and requirements of consciousness in the same sense that the postures of Hatha Yoga or the techniques of meditation influence the flow of energies and reflect back along the beam of consciousness various aspects of consciousness which can assist and harmonize a particular part with the whole.

With the right use of structure and the willingness to make consciousness ready for change, the reality of a situation and the Truth underlying it can be revealed. In this way, the true nature in Man with a heightened awareness of spirit centered in the ONE can become a vehicle or a signpost for others to find the direction within themselves.

*See "The Rise of the Phoenix" by Christopher Hills, published by University of the Trees Press.

INDIVIDUAL CHOICE AND UNIVERSAL GUIDANCE

The only thing that binds man to the chain of events, to time and to the karmic cycles of cause/effect, pleasure/pain, life/death, is the inability to change reactions and disturbances into non-action (silence) and to turn non-action into meaningful work from within. When hearing is turned into the power of listening, and looking into the power of seeing, then evolution can take its natural course, observed by the SELF that sees all, and experienced by the self that accepts the role it plays in the cosmic scheme as a whole, with the awareness that both are ONE and the same in the state of pure consciousness. Duality, which had previously seemed to work against growth, becomes complementary to it and necessary for creation to exist. In the state of pure consciousness, there is no need to hold onto creation since, with the attainment of all and an awareness of an eternal blissful existence, why should the Being be in need of creation. To the liberated, the choice is there; to the unliberated there is no choice if he wishes to live in total freedom. As a person is freed of attachment he is no longer tied to the effects of karma. Action is then not a need but a joy from which he deisres nothing but to give of himself. If there is a wanting, a desire unfulfilled, then there is a pressure of time, and the pleasure/pain, life/death cycles have their effect, whereas if life is lived with the joy of living -- full stop! -- then it does not matter whether the life is on the earthly plane, in spirit, or whatever, the joy is there.

One way to experience this joy is to live in the here and now, moment to moment, enjoying the presence of life all around. If one is out in the country, - Fine! - if one is in the town, - Fine! - if one is sitting in meditation, - Fine! - In all situations there can be the feeling of God's presence, the feeling that this is me and I have the choice to add something to this situation or to just

296

enjoy being in it. If I don't enjoy being in it, then it is a part of myself that I don't like and all I have to do is to look at it from another angle and either change the thought or change the situation, which is ultimately the same thing. The whole of creation is an endless stream of thoughts in the universal mind of God.

To the attached person it is in the process of changing thoughts, feelings and situations that problems begin to arise. Once the realization comes that any limitations in changing things are imposed by ourself, then we can start to develop the willingness to change and, at the same time, the faith that all things are possible. Sometimes a change can be instantaneous and other times it may take a systematic step-by-step approach with patient perseverence to completely master the obstacle that is in the way to experiencing a new state of consciousness. When difficult things become easy, growth has taken place.

The important thing to realize in changing is that the change is already there in the consciousness; it just needs attunement to it. The state of pure consciousness is already present. It is a sense of time that puts it at a distance. Desire and the sense of time do, however, have their place in realizing one's true nature. By moving consciousness through the levels we gain experience and a greater understanding of the ONE.

This last effect can be seen taking place at the chemical level in the way that a phosphor particle in a material gives the material the ability to absorb light and jump from the phosphorescent state of wanting to absorb light, to luminescence - absorbing and radiating that light on a new energy level.

The state of pure consciousness contains no-thing as it is pure, and yet all things are in it for it is the essence of all. In darkness or with closed eyes one may see nothing, but by vibrating the energy of silence, images can be formed and that vibrating energy can become light. With concentration upon that vision produced by the light reflected from it, the images receive more light and can become more vivid and "real". Try it and see. Out of the darkness (void) of God's silence, perhaps God also concentrates on some image and perhaps it becomes "real" by "letting there be light" to the extent that he becomes totally involved in it. As the image becomes more "real", the one who imagines and the subject of the imagination may become confused as to who is who. Is that what God is doing? If so, how does he become clear (pure) again?

When white (transparent) light is concentrated at a point with sufficient power, it becomes a spot of white light. Continue and the spot of white becomes black. If we "throw" sufficient light on our own self-image, as in the case of the phosphorized particle above, could it be then that our image of reality will change back to a void of no content? Will we then see the "light" of no consciousness? If we see this, what will God see? And who is God, anyway?

If you want to know the answer to this ONE, ask no one but yourSELF. If you find out the answer to this ONE, don't tell anyone; keep it to yourSELF.

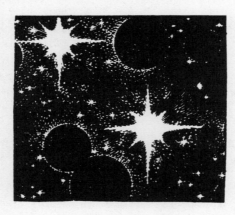

SUMMARY AND EPILOGUE

THE NUCLEAR EVOLUTION APPROACH
TO HATHA YOGA

The title of this book could have been "The Nuclear Evolution Approach To Hatha Yoga. The application of the teachings of Nuclear Evolution (or "Hills' Theory of Consciousness") to the practice of Hatha Yoga speeds up the process of balancing psychophysical energy on all levels and brings the body, mind and soul more rapidly into alignment with the True Self. Yoga is then taken beyond the practice stage to the actualizing of it into everyday living.

For thousands of years now the postures of Hatha Yoga have been practiced for their physiological benefits and as a means of gaining control over the physical body. Some people have taken their practice a state further by studying the psychological reactions and disturbances in the consciousness while moving into an asana (body position) and during the holding of a posture for some time. By observing and altering the states of mind during the practice of postures, it is possible to bring reactions and disturbances under control and to become aware of the nature and conditioning of the soul that causes such effects in the consciousness. Those conscientious aspirants who have focused their search to the deeper levels are able to see the spiritual significance of body positioning, mind processing and soul searching by the light of the True Self, who evolves through these various vibratory channels yet encompasses the whole in a conscious, two-way ingoing and outgoing spiralling of cosmic energy.

The syllables HA and THA of Hatha Yoga refer to these spirals of outgoing energy (HA) and ingoing energy (THA). They are experienced subjectively by an expressive and a receptive nature respectively. The spontaneous creation, maintenance and transformation of life patterns which emanate from these natural spirals

299

of pure life energy on a microcosmic and a macrocosmic scale can be sensed in the body by the yogi who learns to observe from the still Nuclear Center of Being within. He can listen to the vibrations of consciousness on all levels as one whole; that is, with nothing separating the experiencer from the experienced or the observer from the observed.

When these spirals of energy are balanced on all levels, yoga (union with the Source) results and the Self sees the Self clearly, reflecting and experiencing itself as one with the ONE.

The symbols following show the ingoing energy field of consciousness (a); the outgoing energy field (b); and the combined effect in the Symbol of Nuclear Evolution (c), as drawn by Christopher Neave and improved by Regan Power for Christopher Hills' explanation of his theory of consciousness.

THE INGOING SPIRAL OF CONSCIOUSNESS

THE OUTGOING SPIRAL OF CONSCIOUSNESS

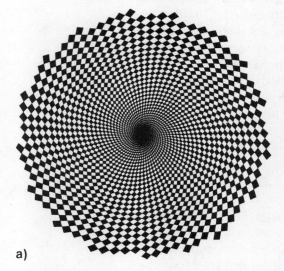

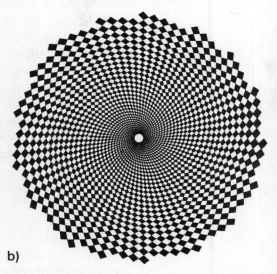

a)

The energy field of the receptive void, which draws into itself that which is of itself.

b)

The energy field of the creative heaven, which radiates its own light into the world of nature.

THE SYMBOL OF NUCLEAR EVOLUTION

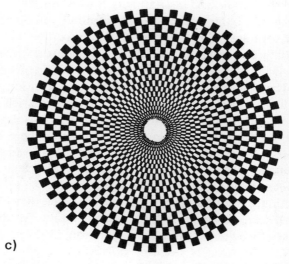

c)

The still center is surrounded by a deep vortex of changing patterns of spiritual energy. This symbol represents the seer's eye, its iris and its retina, the replication of the Spiritual Sun and the cosmic nucleus.

In the human body there are seven spinal nervous centers and seven endocrine glands which relate to seven cosmic energy centers produced by the interaction of the ingoing and outgoing fields of energy with the light of consciousness. Nuclear Evolution explains this process and describes the effects of the seven centers with respect to resonant vibratory color levels and corresponding psychological drives in the human personality.

In certain of the asanas of Hatha Yoga, a specific positioning of the body directs an energy flow into one of the seven centers, called chakras, which then opens it up to an outflow of the essence consciousness seated within that chakra. This happens however, only when the shaping of the body, attitude of mind and openness of the soul are aligned correctly. The resultant balance of ingoing and outgoing spirals of consciousness in that particular chakra then effects an evolution of consciousness. This is because in the process of evolution, the individual consciousness becomes resonant with the universal pattern of consciousness and the two aspects are integrated as one. In this state of oneness there is no separation between a positioning of the body and the creation of a corresponding effect on other levels of consciousness, including the effect that such a relative patterning of consciousness has on a group situation, a national character trait or a planetary system. All things are seen to be motivated by a common Life Principle. For example, upright standing postures create a vertical structure which encourages an aspiring quality in consciousness. Tall buildings can have the same effect. A group with high-minded aims and good ethics influences these tendencies in one. Knowing this at a deep level gives an insight into the understanding of the mechanism of the particular chakra that is concerned with this type of energy.

Every posture represents a mental attitude, a spiritual quality and an aspect of the Self. A presentation of shape, form and nature in consciousness aligns the expression of some aspect of the Self with the reflection of it back to the Self. When there is no misalignment, direct perception takes place and pure consciousness illumines the soul.

In shape there is a structure composed of lines, which symbolize the male aspect of consciousness. In the human body the skeleton of bones provides the framework for shape. The shaping of the structure by the movement of energy around it supports and encourages its stature with form, the female aspect. The flesh of the body provides the supporting energy of form. The way in which energy is formed around structure describes the inner nature of the artist and in the performance of a posture, this can be seen in the texture and stretching of the skin. In the true marriage of shape, form and nature with the True Self, the spirit enlightens and enlivens the whole with a natural upliftment of the consciousness. The effect in the consciousness of the doer is to do without feeling there is any effort in doing.

In order to find out how the alignment of self with Self can take place in a posture, we need only to look at the natural phenomena of the physiological mechanism of the body to see how structure, form and balance apply. As an example, take Trikonasana, the Triangle pose:

Diagram 15.2.

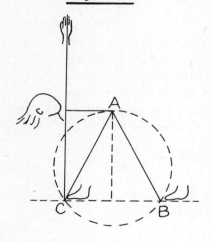 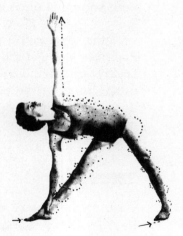

When the triangle A, B, C is made equilateral and the spine is horizontal to the ground, then the vertical arms touch the foot to create a perfectly symmetrical shape. This resonates with the mental vibration of firmness and the spiritual vibration of perserverance. When one is conscious of these qualities in the position and at ease within, then a direct reflection of Truth feeds back to the Self, a direct knowing of attunement between what is manifested and what is unmanifested by the SELF.

In being conscious of the natural spiralling of energies in the body, the correct shaping of the body can be encouraged and the realization of oneness with these universal energies can be realized. The photograph above shows the spirals around the body in Trikonasana.

The spirals as shown above can be similarly sensed in all postures. By a suitable choice of postures, it is possible to focus energy into each chakra in turn. Some postures are in tune with the ingoing spiral of consciousness while there are others which are in tune with the outgoing spiral of consciousness.

In the Nuclear Evolution method of Hatha Yoga Practice, the natural spirals of ingoing and outgoing energy are stimulated by specific postures in a specific order. Some of these specific postures follow and when done in the order A-N, they provide for a balance of ingoing and outgoing energies on all levels of consciousness.

Diagram 15.3.

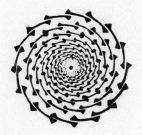

Postures which stimulate the outgoing (yang) effect are:

A	Red	Utthitta Parsvakonasan (Lateral Angle Pose)
M	Orange	Utthitta Trikonasan (Triangle Pose)
C	Yellow	Parivrtta Trikonasan (Reverse Triangle Pose)
K	Green	Bhujangasan (Cobra Pose)
E	Blue	Rajakapotanasan (Pigeon Pose)
I	Indigo	Vrschikasan (Scorpion Pose)
G	Violet	Adho Mukha Vrikshasan (Handstand Pose)

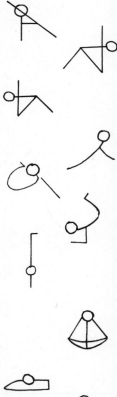

Postures which stimulate the ingoing (yin) effect are:

N	Red	Baddha Konasan (Cobblers Pose)
B	Orange	Paschimottanasan (Head-to-toe Pose)
L	Yellow	Ardha Matseyendrasan (Spinal Twist Pose)
D	Green	Chakrasan (Wheel Pose)
J	Blue	Sarvangasan (Shoulderstand Pose)
F	Indigo	Karnapidasan (Broken Plough Pose)
H	Violet	Sirshasan (Headstand Pose)

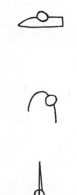

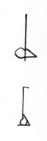

Other aids to posture practice that come through the teachings of Nuclear Evolution are:

a) The visualization of the center symbol radiating from each chakra center as the appropriate posture is being practiced.

b) Toning a note that is found to center the consciousness in the chakra that is being focused into by a posture.

c) Feedback by the body as to possible areas of growth — each area of the body relates to a particular chakra energy and color level.

Feet and legs	Red
Pelvic Girdle	Orange
Navel	Yellow
Chest	Green
Neck	Blue
Face	Indigo
Top of Head	Violet

Whenever there is a difficulty or a pain in an area of the body when in a posture, this indicates a need to look at the psychological and spiritual problems in that area and to deal with them at the level in which they are at, as well as continuing to practice the posture.

Seeing the way round to doing a posture physically by say, doing other postures relating to other chakras first, indicates also the possible route to take by mental attitudes and a study of the personality traits in those areas as described in Nuclear Evolution.

Remember that when the body is seen as a reflection of the mind and soul and also as a miniature planet or universe, then wherever the consciousness is focused, one may also see the cause and effect principle at work on other levels. When this is realized, true oneness can be integrated onto all levels and evolution from the Nuclear Self actualized.

INDEX

A

Activity -- 55
Actualization -- 212
Adaptability -- 70
Analysis -- 100,114
Apana -- 126, 148, 166
Asanas -- 41,42,43,44,61,
62,79,80
Atoms -- 35
Attunement -- 212
Authority -- 139, 162, 259
Awareness -- 68, 214

B

Backbends -- 79, 234
Bhagavad Gita -- 286
Bible -- 257
Body areas -- 71, 105, 142, 151
Brahman -- 286
Breath --
 Shakti -- 224
 Shiva -- 224
Breathing --
 approach to -- 92, 167
 cleansing -- 152, 168
 effects of -- 92, 168
 ratios -- 149
 types of -- 168
Buddha -- 271

C

Center -- 27, 300
Chakras -- 123, 124, 179, 219
Chakrasana -- 235
Chanting -- 193, 270, 287
Christ Consciousness -- 29, 275
Circulation -- 70, 71

Color -- 104, 107, 169, 183, 245, 253, 279, 301

Concentration -- 159
Conceptual -- 112
Conscious -- 214
Consciousness -- 123
 essence of -- 240
 focusing of -- 280
 functions of -- 67, 86
 laws of -- 23, 27, 32, 67,
 86, 240
 levels of -- 30, 106, 160, 169,
 251
 maps of -- 112, 140, 253
 planes of -- 176, 178, 281
 pure -- 31, 274, 279
 states of -- 201, 214
Contractability -- 70
Counterpose -- 114
Creation -- 197, 200,201
Creative Conflict -- 145
Cleansing -- 168
Course in Yoga -- 37
Cosmic -- 239
Cycle -- 35, 52, 115, 215

D

Delusion -- 231
Desire -- 130, 140
Devotion -- 138
Direct --
 experience -- 241
 perception -- 185, 241
Direction -- 78, 94, 228
Discipline -- 87, 88
Diversity -- 14, 290
Divination -- 255
Dorje -- 269
Drives --
 psychological -- 105, 109,
 183

NEGATIVE IONS: A NEW DEVELOPMENT IN HOME ECOLOGY

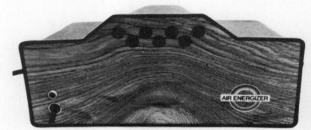

SYSTEM FOUR

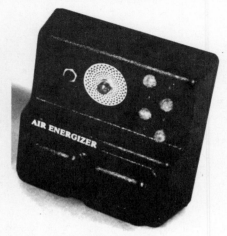

SYSTEM THREE

Recent research shows that tiny electrically charged air particles called negative ions can protect you against air pollution, help put more oxygen in your blood, improve your breathing, promote mental alertness and enhance natural vitality.

Few people know that often the very environment they live and work in can be robbing them of vital energy. The "invisible robber" is the imbalance of negative to positive ions in the air you breathe. And the greatest imbalance is often found in our cities, offices and homes.

Researcher Dr. Felix Sulman of Hebrew University in Israel has shown that too many positive ions cause irritability, tiredness and if too much in excess, nausea, migraine, and eye disorders. An abundance of negative ions however, promotes vitality.

Our own group of researchers here have confirmed that in an atmosphere charged with negative ions less sleep is needed, greater mental alertness is achieved, and more vitality is felt. Negative ions will also help clear rooms of dust and smoke as they quickly attach themselves to these positively charged particles and make them sink to the earth.

Unfortunately our civilized lifestyles often mean we have to live in areas with abnormally high concentrations of positive ions. Air heaters, fluorescent lights, electric appliances, computers, air conditioners, freeways, TV sets and many other things we consider necessary are often sources of positive ions.

What can be done about this problem? Negative ions are more concentrated in wooded areas, near waterfalls, in the mountains, by beaches and swift streams and where there is fresh sunlight. However, most of us can't live in such settings and need a practical alternative. This is why we've designed our AIR ENERGIZERS.

These electronic AIR ENERGIZERS will feed trillions of negative ions into your depleted air and revitalize it into healthy air.

In the past four years we have become recognized as pioneers in this field by knowledgeable individuals and independent research labs have reported the quality and superiority of our units. We are proud to be able to offer you a piece of equipment that we are getting so much positive feedback on.

If you're interested, order one of our units now and we'll ship immediately. Once you receive it turn it on and feel the cool ion "wind" coming off the emitters. Try it out for a few days and see how alert and refreshed you feel. If you are dissatisfied in any way return it in 10 days for a full cash refund.

YOUR CHOICE OF TWO TOP QUALITY UNITS!
System Three: Rugged and durable with a heavy duty transformer. Solid State. $139.00 plus $5.50 shipping and handling.
System Four: A touch of class. Handsomely designed desk model complements any room. Solid State. $159.00 plus $4.00 shipping.
You Can Charge It! ☐ Master Charge ☐ Visa

Card # _____ Card expiration date: _____

Name _____
(Please print)

Signature _____

UNIVERSITY OF THE TREES PRESS, Box 644
Boulder Creek, CA 95006 (408) 338-3855

Distributorships still available in some cities.

Publishers of practical spiritual guides, scientific books and correspondence courses

INTO MEDITATION NOW: A COURSE OF STUDY, by Christopher Hills $45.00 ★
This cost covers the registration and introduction to the comprehensive three-year course of study that enables you to make the philosophy of Nuclear Evolution a reality in your direct experience. Write for more details.

MEDITATING WITH CHILDREN, by Deborah Rozman   5.95 ★
The first of its kind! A delightful teaching book that brings the great art and science of meditation and conscious evolution to children of all ages, this workbook is being used in classrooms throughout the country as a nonreligious text in centering and awareness development.

EXPLORING INNER SPACE, by Christopher Hills and Deborah Rozman   9.95 ★
Our most popular book. For adults and children. Easy directions for 80 experiences to expand sensory perception, social contact, energy awareness, love, memory, intuition, imagination, and "The Force" within you.

SUPERSENSONICS, by Christopher Hills   15.00 ★
The Diviner's bible and encyclopedia that describes actual methods of measuring psychic electricity (prana) and the ways ancient masters and civilizations arrived at advanced knowledge of perception which shows you how to communicate with plants, crystals, atoms, Cosmic Intelligences or your true Self. A mind-bending book.

ALIVE TO THE UNIVERSE, by Robert Massy   9.95 ★
A physicist explains Supersensonics in simple layman's language, and gives step-by-step instructions on how to divine for lost objects, people, water, minerals, health, etc. Your vast potential for multi-dimensional awareness awaits unfolding through this book. An illustration a page.

ENERGY, MATTER AND FORM, by P. Allen, R. Smith and A. Bearne   9.95 ★
Three consciousness researchers provide a dynamic workbook for those ready to test the bounds of their consciousness. It shows how to perform experiments for unfolding extra-ordinary dimensions of experience. This comprehensive text presents extensive information and insight into the human aura, psychic energy centers, kundalini, psychotronics, electrophotography, divining, acupuncture research, radionics, holography, black holes, pyramid energies and the Creative Imagination.

RAYS FROM THE CAPSTONE, by Christopher Hills   4.95 ★
After 20 years of in depth research into pyramid energies, we now have a book which contradicts many fantasies about meditation and pyramid power, shows the positive and negative uses of pyramid energies and explains the Pi-ray orgone accumulator coffer, a "natural" power dynamo invented by the author which allows you to use pyramid energy safely for growing healthier plants, changing emotional states, zapping yourself with energy, and purifying consciousness.

SUPERSENSONIC INSTRUMENTS OF KNOWING, by Christopher Hills   1.95 ★
This book provides instructions on the use of various Supersensonics tools, rods, pendulums, etc., in a complete catalog of biofeedback instruments and their uses.

HILLS' THEORY OF CONSCIOUSNESS, by Robert Massy   7.95 ★
A student of a master of consciousness describes his own development in a group of 15 selected students of Nuclear Evolution. This book contains simplified accounts of inspired research of the actual structure of consciousness and its many drives which physicist Massy believes will dominate the next 500-1,000 years of man's history.

HANDBOOK OF NATURAL HEALING, by Michael Ash, M.D.   2.95 ★
Dr. Ash gives a few key principles you'll need to know in order to heal, such as: How long and how often do you heal? The healer and the doctor. Can natural healing do any harm? The life energy field. Positive imagination. Must a patient have faith to be healed?

All prices subject to change without notice.

THE RISE OF THE PHOENIX, by Christopher Hills   14.95 ★

Throughout time the mythical Phoenix has symbolized the death of old values and the dawning of a New Age. Christopher Hills has written this book at a time in our history when the planet is besieged by raging conflicts at all levels of life.

Rise of the Phoenix shows what we can do to give birth to a new social, economic, political, and spiritual order. With vivid photographs throughout, it portrays the world as a stage for power cliques and selfish interests that destroy freedom. The book studies the qualities and mistakes of great leaders and their effect on history.

Over the past 25 years Dr. Hills has established experimental communities around the world serving as models of self-government and personal evolution. This highly readable account of the positive and negative forces at work inside all people opens up a new view of how we can change human destiny.

Your Electro-Vibratory Body, by Victor Beasley, PhD. $9.95 ★

This book contains a selection of research from the world's foremost pioneers who look at the human body as a collection of atoms and molecules whirling around in space. They see the effects of one's auric field extending far beyond the physical body. They show how your mood, personality and health are affected and governed by magnetic and electric fields, positive and negative ions, light and colors, and even the thoughts of others. This information, once regarded as occult, is now the focus of research by M.D.'s and Ph.D.'s.

Nuclear Evolution: Discovery of the Rainbow Body, by Christopher Hills

Deluxe paperback $12.95   Hardback library edition $18.95 ★

This book is perhaps the most authoritative look at the evolutionary potentials of the human race ever published. Light is the theme of the book: that the human personality is formed from waves and pulses of light. Humans and other animals and objects eat light, and the human mind is a black hole that absorbs light, then emits it as the rainbow body. A masterpiece in consciousness research.

Food From Sunlight, by Christopher Hills   paperback $14.95 ★

The Japanese have known since 1917 that successful harvesting of algae would produce infinite amounts of food from air, light and water. Failure to do so prompted in 1959 the Japanese newspaper article, *Chlorella Algae, the Manna from Heaven, is a Twentieth Century Myth.* But in 1963 Spirulina algae was discovered and, over the next ten years, brought manna from heaven to a reality. In Japan it now sells ounce for ounce the same price as gold, due to its nutritional values and rejuvenation properties.

May You Live in Health, by Aaron Friedell, M.D.   paperback $3.95 ★

After meeting 80-year old Aaron Friedell, you would want to buy his book—a guide to effective health habits. His system is the result of forty year's practice as a physician and researcher on increasing the vigor of the human body and obtaining peace of mind. Although practical, Dr. Friedell's book has some amazing technical data explained simply.

The Politics of God, by Dr. Hugh J. Schonfield $9.95 ★

The author of *The Passover Plot* does it again! In this book his aim is to show that Christianity as practiced today is not identical with what Jesus of Nazereth or his immediate followers taught but represents a deviation from their beliefs. This book picks up the ancient Messianic idea and gives it a modern application bringing together once again the essential faith of Jews and Christians.

Journey Into Light, by Ann Ray   Paperback $7.95 ★

Journey Into Light is a timely book, for it is the story of a woman who, in her late 30's, leaves her husband and her established place in an academic community and goes in search of her true Self. Her spiritual commitment, tested in a karmic sexual situation, is a powerful statement of Nuclear Evolution, not in theory but as a living human experience. A book for anyone in search of love. **All prices subject to change without notice.**

RUMF ROOMPH YOGA

A unique series of spiritual teachings on cassette tape.

The teachings in this series called *Rumf Roomph Yoga* were first presented to students of Christopher Hills during the first half of 1975. Based on the Yoga Sutras of Patanjali, these teachings and exercises have always been given orally because their powerful vibration could not be communicated via the written word. What you, the sincere listener, receive while meditating with the tapes is the equivalent of an initiation into higher levels of consciousness usually only possible in the presence of a guru. Here that presence is evoked from within your being over and over every time you listen to a tape and join in the exercises.

Because of the intense building-block nature of the series *Rumf Roomph Yoga* tapes are available only in sequence. You may purchase the whole series at once or a portion, so long as that portion is in order (i.e. #1-2, 1-3, 1-4, etc.). Or you may like to order them one at a time. These are all practical, consciousness-expanding sessions!

Session One
GETTING ROOMPH INTO MEDITATION

This tape begins with a powerful guided meditation in which you withdraw consciousness from your body to one point in the Ajna chakra (psychic center). Then you radiate it out through space, expanding your idea of self. This is a meditation for realizing the nature of Brahman (God) and for finding out how big is Big. Christopher then talks on the nature of mindstuff and the process of identification. How does mind color your perceptions? How can we come to see everything as it truly is? *1½ hrs., $9.00.*

Session Two
DEVELOPING SPIRITUAL MUSCLES

Several exercises for 1) Developing superconscious awareness and growing more brain cells. 2) Basic Buddhist practice of mindfulness, mindlessness and total openness. When mind is pure and mindless there is nothing for it to cling to. Then it becomes all-objective which is voidness, shunyata. This is not a passive state but a dynamic mind-transcendence. 3) Samyama—concentration, expansion and identification in oneness. By doing samyama knowledge arises of mindstuff and of otherness. 4) Cobra Snake dance done to chanting for purification of mindstuff. Tuning into the merudanda at the center of the spine which manufactures cerebro-spinal fluid, the quality of which determines what you will experience of the universe. 5) Control of sound—Nada Banda. The union of the psychological and physiological forces with the vibrating OM, Nadam or supersonic sound current. Body is transformed into life current, respiration is stopped and finer forces awakened. *1hr. 40 min., $11.00.*

Session Three
SHIVA-SHAKTI ENERGY FLOW

The tantric union of opposites. A tantra asana where Shiva (male) flows continuously to Shakti (female) and ordinary sexual energy is transmuted into new energy. Individual exercises as well as Shiva-Shakti dance with a partner. *2 hrs., $12.00.*

Session Four
CONTROLLING THE CHAKRA FORCES

The ego is made from mindstuff which is luminous but not self-luminous. The Self which sees through the mind is like the sun, mind is like the moon. Understanding the relationship between the senses, the mind and Self as Pure Consciousness. Consciousness and light as One. Whatever is not happening out there is because it's not happening in here, inside us. Understanding the chakra forces and purifying them by looking into our reactions. *1 hr. 50 min., $11.00*

All prices subject to change without notice.

Session Five
RADICALIZING THE EGO

The Self sense arises from recognition of expansion of the Universal Ego. Exercises for: 1)Learning to use your body as a feedback machine. 2) Meditation on the Center Symbol Mandala for the experience of primary light of consciousness. Sending and receiving the white light of prana. The entire environment experienced as a feedback of consciousness. 3) Meditation for going through the Center of the symbol, the crown chakra, and the cosmic penetration of the ego. *1 hr. 10 min., $9.00.* Nuclear Evolution center symbol a must for this . . . $1.95.

Session Six
GETTING CONTROL OF THE EGO

In order to control ego we have to pull consciousness out of the unreal images of reality. The superconscious Self punishes when you let the ego get on the throne. Going deeper into total openness where there is no otherness. Selflessness as no separation between the knower and the object known, self and God. Surrendering your defenses and becoming psychologically naked in communication with the One and others. The Tree of Knowledge and the Tree of Life explained as the knowledge of separation vs. the Oneness. How to reverse the flow of energy from the senses towards the spirit. *1hr. 45min., $11.00.*

Session Seven
EXPANDING THE SELF SENSE AND BURSTING THE EGO BUBBLE

Kaivalyam as the actionless action of liberation. Meditation on Total Openness using the Center Symbol. Recognizing the Self everywhere. Mudra exercise for seeing the intense light of the spiritual eye within. Om chanting for Cosmic Initiation. *1 hr. 10 min., $9.00.*

Session Eight
EGO, SUPERCONSCIOUS, MIND AND IMAGINATION

An intensely deep and concentrated discussion on these four aspects of our being. You will learn to recognize and experience their workings in your own consciousess and how they interact to affect and condition each other. More on Nada Banda and Om chanting as a means of transcendence. *1 hr., $8.00.*

Session Nine
MEDITATION AND BREATH CONTROL

Exercises for doing yogic bandas (banda means control) for using sexual energies for higher purposes. Thus the inner energies become a potent force for finding the One. When ego directs the sexual energies for selfish gratification it brings false satisfaction. When it causes the energies to fly upward and unite with the universal energy, fulfillment is found. Controlling internal and external breathing and chanting Om as the highest breathing exercise. *1hr. 35 min. $10.00.*

Session Ten
UNDERSTANDING PURE CONSCIOUSNESS

An introductory tape to our three-year meditation course in Direct Perception. An explanation of how to use Buddhist mandalas, experiencing the essence of Christ's teachings and dissolving the ego. Christopher answers questions from students, and the University of the Trees residents share their insights. *1 hr., $8.00.*

Session Eleven
PRACTICING THE PRESENCE OF GOD

Keeping an inner silent prayer going through all activity. This constantly tunes you in a form of continuous worship. By practicing the Presence in your own self you are able to tune into it in all selves. The presence is a bliss disturbed only by self limitation. Christopher talks about the mind traps that block the Presence and stop the flow of grace. Learn to listen to your life situation. Exercise with a group for releasing hang-ups with others, especially sexual. *1 hr. 35 min., $10.00.*

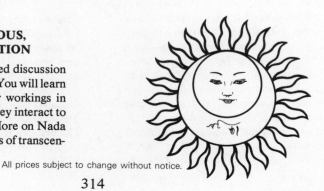

All prices subject to change without notice.

314

Session Twelve
VALIDATION OF YOGIC METHODS OF KNOWING

How do you know what you don't know? Getting beneath the words to essence knowledge. Recognizing the difference between knowledge which is learned and knowledge gained by direct perception. Do you really know what you think you know? In direct knowing the subject and object must be considered as one. Many psychics are deluded so intuitions still must be tested. Empirical experience has to be validated as meaningful. Look to the real manifestation of any guru. There is no truth that can be seen except from the viewpoint of the knower. What is true for you is true from your own viewpoint. Exercise in the group situation to gauge the quality of detachment from ego-centric judgement. Experiment for washing your mind clear of previous concepts with a partner as your mirror. Taking a journey to a higher life. The Samadhi experience. Seeing the Source and Naked Essence in another. *1hr. 45 min., $11.00.*

Session Thirteen
GROUP EXERCISE FOR DISSOLVING OUR SEPARATED SELF

Complete samyama: concentration for one-pointedness, expansion to include all dissolution of separated self in samadhi. Doing samyama on anything—becoming one with objects, with our own psychic process and with others. How you can transmit Pure Being and see its reflection work through others unconsciously. *1 hr. 50 min., $11.00.*

Session Fourteen
CONTACTING THE TREE OF LIFE AND THE TREE OF KNOWLEDGE

If you identify with the mindstuff you get trapped because that's past karma. Learning to welcome suffer-ing when it happens as a teacher, and being true to your self. Transmitting Pure Being to another as yourself. Meditation with another person. Sitting knee to knee you meditate on death. You die and enter the Garden of Eden and look into the eyes of the other. You see the Soul, the Tree of Life, and you look through the body-senses, the Tree of Knowledge. Surrendering to the great evolutionary intelligence in trust to give you what you need. *1hr., $8.00.*

Session Fifteen
EVOLUTIONARY GROUP INTERACTION

The love seat exercise. This is a group medita-tionneeding two persons or more. Here we do samyama on each person in turn. The whole group tunes to each being and gives feedback. Comments are recorded as well as the name of the person who made them. When everyone has had their turn this group evaluates how much was a projection, a semi-projection or a direct perception. This exercise is the introduction for working directly on the ego in a group situation. Through the eyes of each other we expand our vision of ourself. *1 hr., $8.00.*

Session Sixteen
CREATIVE CONFLICT

Mastering self-intoxication with self-saturation. The key to bliss is to stop identifying with your needs, desires and wish fulfillments. Whatever you see, experience – your internal show – that is the true quality of your manifested self. Your situation is what you have not mastered. Work-ingtogether for self-mastery and discovering the Self in others. What is the manifested situation of our life trying to teach us? This tape includes the principles and rules of Creative Conflict, a western form of yoga, which is a major part of the group work at the University of the Trees. Applying these principles makes group work penetrating, creative, and brings group consciousness. *2 hrs., $12.00.*

Session Seventeen
BECOMING A SOUL MIRROR

The Nuclear group as a cosmic mirror. How to use a group as a feedback machine for penetrating the ego and gaining group consciousness. You levitate and radiate into the boundless universe so there is no inward-reflecting consciousness. Meditation on the Divine Craziness. Creating a free flow of Akasha through the walls, stars, and beyond the idea of empty space, to a state where nothing disturbs. Your mind no longer reacts to anyone or anything because it goes through all things. You dissolve your programs of how you see yourself and relate to others in this new state. We become cosmic soul mirrors for each other, watching for what disturbs us as the key to what we have to work on to get to our deep karmas. *2 hrs, $12.00.*

All prices subject to change without notice.

Session Eighteen
ANAHATA NADAM

Chanting through the heart center you enter the nadam, the Om, the supersonic sound current which is inside and outside. You enter Saguna Brahman, the state of mindless radiant energy rw1 where the gunas or creative forces are controlled.

By concentrating on Nadam you can experience Nirguna Brahman where the gunas that create the manifested world disappear in Pure Consciousness. *1 hr., $8.00.*

Session Ninteen
QUESTIONS AND ANSWERS

Group discussion of the *Rumf Roomph Yoga* series experiences to date. Many questions are answered. The gaps in individual's consciousness are explained and considered. Typical insights, concerns and thoughts are expressed, some of which you will probably have in your own mind. *1 hr. 35 min., $10.00.*

Session Twenty
MAHAVIDEHA

Super-penetration of the mindstuff of Self and others. This is the exercise for the great penetration of our desires, motives and identification with personality. The first step seems like a hypnosis because you still look at everyone separately when you come down. This is an imaginary state of Videha. Super-penetration is the real thing where the real relation between soul and personality can manifest in you. Here you don't just listen to the words but manifest them too. Mahavideha can only happen through Samyama. By doing Mahavideha we can enter into the bodies of students and help them to understand their confusion. All desires are realized as instruments of the One, pulling us along the path of Nuclear Evolution. The double-acting effect of light and consciousness is explained. Brahman Consciousness is distinguished as Absolute penetration wherever there ojectless consciousness. *1hr. 30 min., $10.00.*

Rumf Roomph Yoga is derived from the mantram
Rumf Roomph Drivenam Swa

Session Twenty-One
BALANCING LEVITY AND GRAVITY

Master the chakra forces and control the gunas, creative forces. Realizing the nature of the True Self by exploring the 7 levels of consciousness in the Nuclear group. An outline of the levels in the group situation and learning to recognize the levels as they appear through your own actions and words and in others. The importance of the Nuclear Group for seeing your blind spots and intensifying the evolutionary momentum. *1 hr. 55 min., $12.00.*

Session Twenty-Two
DISCOVERING YOUR KARMA

Advanced exercises for awakening Shakti force and increasing the kundalini flow. The nature of karmas and how to reveal your true karma. Surrendering to the Cosmic Lover who sits inside as your true guru, your own true Self. The marriage of Shiva and Shakti in Brahma Consciousness. Making decisions as to what your real work is, your karma. How is your love made visible in selfless service and selfless actions. The joy of service and doing the work for the One. *1 hr., $8.00.*

Session Twenty-Three
PURIFYING THE CHAKRAS

A powerful tool for tuning into the vibrations of the seven chakras and being able to recognize them, work with them and cleanse them through sound and consciousness. Overcoming resistance and inertia. Understanding of the guna forces. Exercise for radiating consciousness through each of your chakras. *1 hr., $8.00.*

Session Twenty-Four
EMBODYING THE AVATAR CONSCIOUSNESS

Awakening within you the Avatar Consciousness. The manifestation of the true Avatar. Discriminating the true avatar from the assumed one. The nature of Powers, siddhis and Pure Consciousness. The nature of the true Messianic consciousness from the deluded one which always refers to itself as the source. How to test ourselves, and what are essential criteria for fulfillment of a Divine Mission. *1 hr., $8.00.*

Rumf being the spirit of life, *Roomph,* the vital force of prana bubbling from the base of the spine and spilling over into the heart as in the rising of kundalini, *Drivenam* meaning the wealth of the universe, total certainty and security which is to go out of the mind into the real self, and *swa* is sweetness or bliss which comes like ambrosia to melt the ego, as a baby does, until the self becomes sweet inside its own self, producing saintliness.

All prices subject to change without notice.

YOGIC METHODS OF LEARNING

Speed Tape Learning Institute of University of the Trees

Foreword by Your Director of Studies

Speed Tape Learning is a new way of absorbing knowledge while you hover between sleep and waking, using a simple cassette or reel to reel tape recorder which is switched on by the student and switches off with the aid of an automatic shut off switch. Speed tape learning is more effective than sleep learning, therefore the student should switch on his tape recorder on retiring and relax completely while listening to the subject to be learned. He will pass on to ordinary sleep without any interference in natural sleep. Sleep is in fact enhanced because of the extra depth which ensues after the tape comes to an end.

First the student plays our conditioning tape which puts him in a special state of consciousness by using yogic techniques of induction. Our founder Christopher Hills was able to read between 25 and 50 books a day by using these methods of training himself to have a photographic memory. You too can use the same methods to cultivate an auditory memory. First the pre-sleep method conditions the student for learning in a two-step process. The material to be learnt is first heard under pre-sleep conditioning and then the following day in a fully conscious state, so that our subconscious mind is already prepared for absorption of the material. The technique is efficient and cumulative so that after a few weeks the memory learning rate is vastly accelerated.

There are many new methods of speed sleep learning, under such names as "suggestology", and in Russia reports of marvelous academic results have been claimed. In America and Britain seminars for learning languages have been given under license from Dr. Lozanov, but actually the phenomenon has been known to yogis for centuries.

If your tape recorder does not have an automatic shut-off switch then you need to buy a time switch or buy a cassette recorder with a shut-off switch, so that you don't have to worry about the machine being on while you sleep. Anxiety about the machine being left on acts as a blockage to subconscious tape-learning.

Is a pillow speaker necessary? Yes, the pillow speaker has been found to present the information at the whisper level so that it is just audible, and the yogis and lamas discovered the whisper technique is more acceptable for the subconscious mind. The Tibetan Book of the Dead was always whispered in the ear. It is also important that you should be totally receptive and not worried about other people hearing your tape recorder noise.

The college offers a 60-minute tape guidance on how to employ the technique on one side and the conditioning pre-sleep on the other. For rapid success this tape should be first purchased with any other of the self-improvement courses and healing tapes. These tapes and equipment are offered in this catalog.

The student needs to have the basic requirements of a tape recorder, a time switch or cassette recorder with autostop, a pillow speaker, and the guidance and conditioning tape. With this basic equipment the student is ready to increase his capacity for learning and cassette recorder with autostop, a pillow speaker, and the guidance and conditioning tape. With this basic equipment the student is ready to increase his capacity for learning and healing.

The tape courses are designed not only as learning of information but as "essence knowledge" which can overcome personality limitations, develop your understanding of problems, and improve relationships. They are given to generally improve your psychic and physical health, and students at the University of the Trees have proved this for themselves. They are dedicated to sharing this unique knowledge of human nature with you.

I myself am a physicist and I am one of those dedicated students of our founder. I can only tell you that this wisdom has transformed my life permanently. I taught speed reading for several years professionally before I came upon these teachings. There is simply no comparison! These teachings communicate essence knowledge which has given me the ability to author several books and edit several more.

Yours sincerely, *Robert E. Massy*   Director of Studies, Speed Learning Institute

Many of us have found that it's one thing to hear spiritual teachings and another to live them. This gap between hearing and doing has its roots in how deeply we've really heard. The essence teachings of Christopher Hills provide practical answers to life's problems. They help you develop greater awareness and greater joy. And this special tape learning method helps you to absorb very deeply the teachings expressed.

If you already have a cassette tape recorder with automatic shut-off then all you need is a pillow speaker and our special conditioning tape to get started. If your recorder doesn't have this important shut-off addition you'll need the above timer to shut off the tape for you or get a recorder that does have a shut-off mechanism.

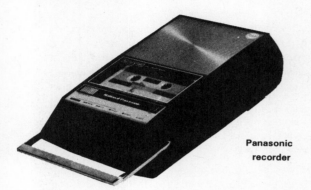

Panasonic recorder

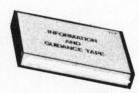

Information and Guidance Tape: Side one of this tape is an introduction to speed tape learning. It explains how to use this method for gaining spiritual knowledge (or learning anything for that matter),. Side two is a guided meditation to put you into yoga nidra or a state of twilight sleep in which you can place knowledge into your subconscious mind. 1 cassette *$8.00 plus $1.00 postage and handling.*

Portable Repeating Timer: Attractive versatile timer has 15 amp capacity for controlling your cassette recorder, appliances, Hi Fi, heaters, etc. Minimum on time, ¼ hour. Maximum off time, 23 ¾ hours. Manual off/on over-ride switch. Color coded trippers. Easy to set time dial has large AM and PM divisions readable even in dim light. *$10.95 plus $2.50 postage and handling.*

Panasonic Player/Cassette Recorder: Sleek portable cassette recorder. AC/Battery operation. Built-in condenser microphone. Pushbutton controls. Easy-Matic circuitry automatically adjusts recording level. Continuous tone control. Fast forward and rewind. Earphone monitor. Solid State. *$39.95. Please add $3.50 for postage and handling.*

Pillow Speaker: This new pillow speaker is a very superior one that contains a high grade unit which gives better intelligibility at lower volumes and its impedance is exactly matched to all tape recorders. The quality of the sound is also good for musical reproduction and therefore you can listen to radio programs etc. in bed. The speaker is best placed just at the side of your pillow. *$3.95 Plus $2.50 postage and handling.*

NAME————————————————————
ADDRESS——————————————————
————————————————————ZIP—————————

Please give street address as these items must be shipped by UPS.

Please send me the items listed below. I have included postage and handling and have enclosed full payment.

Quan.	Description	Price

All prices subject to change without notice.

Sub-Total	
Calif. residents add 6% tax.	
Postage & Handling.	
TOTAL ENCLOSED	

NEW AGE DIVINING INSTRUMENTS

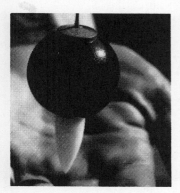

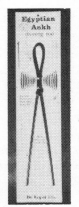

THE AURA PENDULUM PACKAGE ★
Loaded with instructions on how to read auras, the package consists of:
* One *Aura Pendulum* for reading auras,
* One *Rainbow Aura Booklet* which tells how to use the aura pendulum and gives the meanings of seven colors in both positive and negative aspects.
* One *Supersonic Instruments of Knowing* book, a collection of over 25 divining instruments available and how to use them to benefit yourself. **$8.95**

THE EGYPTIAN ANKH DIVINING ROD ★
The Ankh was the Egyptian's "key of life" and was used for divining. Today's technology has provided a high dielectric polymer so that you can find water, minerals, lost objects and a host of other things. **$8.95**

THE POSITIVE ENERGY SENSOR ☐
Now—a new product which emits energy you can actually feel since it is pretuned to life force. This pendulum generates the power of a huge pyramid without the bulk and bother of building one. Carry it in your pocket or purse. Can be used to charge your body with life energy, check nutritional value of foods, detect the negative energy of disease. Contains ample instructions. **$15.00**

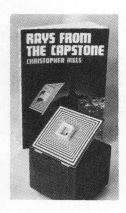

THE PI-RAY COFFER KIT ☐
The most amazing invention to come out of pyramid research. Its awesome powers of "materializing your imaginings" are fully described in the book *Rays From the Capstone* which comes with it. **$83.95**

All the items, books, tapes and instruments on the previous pages are available from UNIVERSITY OF THE TREES PRESS, P.O. Box 644, Boulder Creek, California 95006   (408) 338-3855.

MAILING AND HANDLING CHARGES
Each item has either a ★ or ☐ next to it to indicate its mailing category. Please note which symbol(s) are next to items in your order and use the corresponding column(s) for calculating postage.

FOREIGN
1. Postage & handling rates: $3.00 per item. Your order will be shipped Parcel Post.
2. Book rate is available for $1.50 per book. We are not responsible for lost shipments under book rate.
3. Expect delivery after 5 weeks.
4. Have all checks and money orders stating certified U.S. dollars. **Canadian and Overseas Customers:** Due to changes in U.S. banking policies, we can no longer accept your personal checks unless they are drawn on a U.S. bank. Otherwise, please send Canadian Postal Money Orders in U.S. dollars, U.S. International Postal Money Orders, or bank checks payable on any U.S. bank or banker's agency.

NAME _____

STREET ADDRESS _____

P.O. BOX _____

CITY _____ STATE _____ ZIP _____

PHONE _____

US POSTAGE RATES

Total of Order	★	Tapes ☐	Mixed ★ ☐
0-$4	$1.00	$1.00	$1.00
$4.-$10.	$1.50	$1.50	$1.50
$10.-$15.	$1.75	$1.50	$1.75
$15.-$20.	$2.25	$1.75	$2.00
$20.-$40.	$2.75	$2.50	$3.00
$40.-$80.	$4.25	$2.75	$4.00
$80.-$150.	$6.00	$3.00	$5.00
over $150.	$7.50	$5.00	$7.00

MALCOLM STRUTT, M.A.

Malcolm Strutt was for some years a yoga teacher with the Inner London Education Authority, before starting his own Centre for Conscious Living and becoming Head of Studies at the Centre School for Alternative Education, which is affiliated with the University of the Trees, in California.

Malcolm Strutt's early training and spiritual education was with Paramahansa Yogananda's Self-Realization Fellowship and instruction from Sri B. K. S. Inyengar. In more recent years Dr. Christopher Hills and his teachings of Nuclear Evolution have been Malcolm's main influence and grounding, part of the time at Centre House with The Centre Community and part with University of the Trees of which Dr. Hills is Director. In 1977, Malcolm Strutt was appointed Director of the Irish School of Yoga and is responsible for the training and qualifying of teachers of yoga in Ireland. He is also a Teacher Education Tutor for the British Wheel of Yoga Teacher's Diploma.

A new appointment is the teaching of yoga at Westminster Abbey.

Malcolm Strutt is author of "A Three Stage Course in Yoga". He is also the Initiator and Director of the Centre Yoga Ballet Group, which has given performances at the Commonwealth Institute Theatre and Festival for Mind and Body at Olympia.

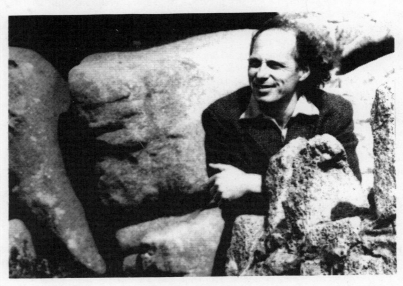